IBS & Colitis

Symptoms, causes, orthodox treatment and
how herbal medicine will help.

Other published and forthcoming titles
in the series include:

Arthritis & Rheumatism

Menopause

Anxiety & Tension

Migraine & Headaches

Asthma & Bronchitis

IBS & Colitis

Jill Wright MNIMH

HERBAL HEALTH

Published in 2001 by
How To Books Ltd, 3 Newtec Place,
Magdalen Road, Oxford OX4 1RE, United Kingdom
Tel: (01865) 793806 Fax: (01865) 248780
email: info@howtobooks.co.uk
www.howtobooks.co.uk

British Library Cataloguing in Publication Data
A catalogue record for this book is available from the British Library

Edited by Diana Brueton
Cover design by Shireen Nathoo Design, London
Produced for How To Books by Deer Park Productions
Designed and typeset by Shireen Nathoo Design, London
Printed and bound in Great Britain
by Bell & Bain Ltd., Glasgow

Herbal Health *is an imprint of*
How To Books

Contents

Preface

What makes you suspect that you have irritable bowel syndrome?

- Have you experienced variable bowel motions – perhaps ranging from constipation to diarrhoea within a short space of time?
- Do you pass more wind downwards (known as flatulence) than you would like?
- Do you suffer from pain in your abdomen on occasions or regularly?

You may find more and more foods 'disagree with you' or you may feel bloated – as though you have eaten a very large meal, even when you last ate hours ago or after quite a small meal.

If you have consulted your GP about symptoms like this, you may have been told you have **IBS – irritable bowel syndrome**. If you are experiencing pain and diarrhoea frequently, passing blood or mucus, losing weight and feeling fatigued, you may have had tests which reveal that you have **colitis**, which is inflammation of the bowel lining, sometimes with ulceration. You may have been told that you have **Crohn's disease** which is a type of ulcerative colitis.

You may have tried various treatments without success

and be looking for an alternative. Herbal medicine is the leading alternative to orthodox drug treatments. It is especially favourable to conditions such as digestive complaints which may have a number of causes and respond well to wholistic treatment.

As a member of the National Institute of Medical Herbalists for ten years I have treated a great number of people with digestive disorders in my clinic. In retail practice I have answered countless queries and given general advice on how to deal with bowel problems. In this book I have written down the answers to questions which are frequently asked. I can offer practical advice on how to treat these conditions, when to consult your doctor and how orthodox as well as herbal medicines work. By reading this book you can:

- Find out
  - the difference between IBS and colitis
  - how to make simple herbal remedies at home
  - how to understand the labels on remedies you buy in shops.
- Get more from visits to hospital consultants and alternative therapists.
- Understand your treatments better.

A brief guide to the processes which happen during digestion will make you more confident in discussing your health with professionals.

The advice contained in this book is meant to be for general use only. If you have a specific medical condition or an allergy, or are taking medication which may affect your use of herbal medicine, you should consult a qualified health care professional such as a doctor or a medical herbalist before starting to use herbal remedies at home.

Jill Wright

1

Understanding IBS and colitis

All about the digestive system

The digestive tract is a tube which consists of mouth, oesophagus, stomach, duodenum, jejunum, ileum, bowel and rectum. Associated organs are the pancreas and liver. You can view the human being as an open ended tube, with:

- two surfaces exposed to the external environment, outside the skin
- and inside, the surface of the digestive tract which is covered in a highly complex secretory lining.

The digestive tract has pockets of immune cells, mucus cells and absorptive cells, which complete the digestive process described below. The whole tract has both lengthwise and circular muscles in its walls which undergo regular contraction and relaxation, independent of brain activity. This type of muscle action is only found in **visceral** muscle, which is also known as smooth muscle, found in the internal organs of the body. The muscles of our body and limbs, which are under conscious control of the brain, are called **somatic**.

The surface of the digestive tract is raised in an immense number of tiny folds called **villi** which make its real extent many times more than if it were a flat surface. These folds also have brush-like extensions all over them which increase the absorptive surface to a fantastic degree.

There are various names for the different segments of the digestive tract. Some writers refer to the **duodenum**, **jejunum** and **ileum** as the small intestine, and the rest as the large intestine. Colon and bowel are names often given to the whole intestine, both large and small. The abbreviation, GIT, stands for **gastro-intestinal tract**. It refers to the whole tract, from mouth to anus. In this book the name **bowel** refers to the tract between stomach and rectum, and the terms **small intestine** and **large intestine** are used to distinguish between the functions of upper and lower bowel.

What happens to food in the mouth?

The moment you smell food, messages are sent to the brain and relayed back to the salivary glands. These produce fluid which contains starch digesting enzymes. This secretion begins the process of digestion and helps the food pass easily down the oesophagus to the stomach. This takes about seven seconds.

What happens to food in the stomach?

The walls of the stomach secrete acid and enzymes which

break down proteins, fats and starch into smaller units. The stomach muscles produce churning movements which help to reduce food to a liquid. This passes through a muscular ring closure – the **sphincter** – into the first part of the small intestine called the **duodenum**.

All of the gastro-intestinal tract is lined with mucus secreting cells, from the mouth to the anus. Mucus has a protective function throughout, especially in the stomach where it has the amazing ability to protect against the hydrochloric acid which is pumped out to digest food. When mucus fails to protect the delicate linings of the GIT, ulcers may form.

What happens to food in the bowel?

As food passes to the duodenum it triggers the release of more digestive enzymes from the pancreas, which take the breakdown of food a bit further. The pancreas also releases bicarbonate to neutralise the stomach acid. This is necessary because the duodenum doesn't have the same degree of mucus protection as the stomach. When food enters the duodenum it causes the gall bladder to release bile, which the liver secreted earlier. This flows into the duodenum where it emulsifies fats so that they can be transported more easily in watery media.

Amino acids from protein, and glucose from starch, along with vitamins and minerals, are absorbed into the bloodstream from the first part of the small intestine, the ileum, by a complex active process in the GIT lining which involves a number of enzymes. These may be destroyed during antibiotic treatment, causing absorption problems. Fat passes into the lymph system and is returned to the blood later.

Surplus protein and starch is stored as fat. Vitamins may be stored or passed out of the body on a daily basis.

All the nutrients we need are absorbed from the small intestine. What remains is called faeces, which consists mainly of bacteria and bile acids. Water and bicarbonate are removed as faeces pass through the large intestine and the rest leaves the body as a semi-solid mass.

What makes a healthy digestive system?

- lymph flow
- blood flow
- regular movement
- good nutrition
- adequate fibre
- relaxed mind.

The whole system is run by nervous impulses to receptors in muscles and secretory cells. These impulses travel in the vagus nerve which connects the brain directly to the GIT. Interconnections with brain centres for emotions allow messages arising from fear, anger, excitement and depression to influence the nervous control of the digestive organs. This is what is called the psychogenic influence in GIT problems. Other nervous impulses travel from the spine and lower brain stem, so we are not in direct control of them. These are known as **autonomic nerves**. They cause secretion and a regular rolling muscle action in the bowel called **peristalsis**. This is most important for the normal function of the digestive system. Fibre is necessary to stimulate peristaltic movement. Disturbances in peristalsis are called motility problems and doctors feel that these are at the heart of IBS.

The autonomic nervous system

The autonomic nerves fall into two groups, oddly called:

1. **sympathetic**
2. **parasympathetic**.

Sympathetic nerves prepare for action and mainly use adrenaline as their chemical messenger. Parasympathetic nerves serve the body in rest and maintenance, and use acetylcholine as their chemical messenger. Strong emotions such as fear and anger cause a greater flow of noradrenaline. Noradrenaline stops secretion and movement in the digestive tract, as well as constricting blood vessels. This explains why stress and anxiety can have such an effect on your digestion – literally reducing movement and absorption. Most people have experienced the dry mouth of anxiety before an exam or an interview. This can become a chronic state of affairs, affecting the secretions of the GIT. The parasympathetic chemical messenger, acetylcholine causes the opposite – increased

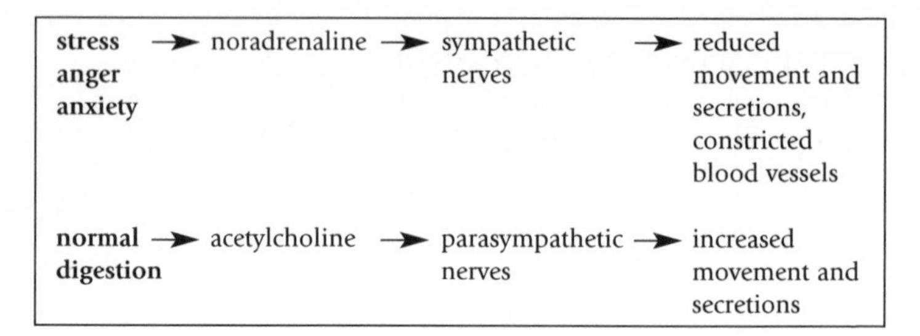

secretions and movement. Doctors use drugs which interfere with acetylcholine to control serious digestive disorders where ulceration is extensive.

The digestive system also relies on efficient blood and lymph flow to pick up nutrients and circulate them. Exercise is the main impetus to lymph flow whereas it is only partly responsible for improvements to blood circulation. Relaxation of the blood vessels may be one of the key elements in blood supplying the digestive tract walls with their own nutrients, as well as carrying them to all parts of the body. Lack of blood supply, known as ischaemia is one of the few events which actually causes pain to be felt in the gut, which isn't well supplied with nervous pain receptors. Some researchers think that constriction of tiny capillaries, which make up a large part of the circulatory system, may be a factor in ulcer development. Noradrenaline, as mentioned above, can cause this during episodes of stress. There may be some chronic recurrence of constriction, which could be called a migraine of the digestive system!

IBS and colitis explained

IBS is not a defined illness but a label given to a group of symptoms when no other pathology (such as inflammation, allergy, infection, ulceration) has been found. The symptoms are found in the lower digestive tract (large intestine). Generally, similar disorders of the upper tract (stomach, oesophagus, duodenum) are known as dyspepsia. The main features of IBS and colitis are:

- intermittent pain
- diarrhoea alternating with constipation
- irritability
- flatulence
- and a type of discomfort which many call bloating.

Diarrhoea

Many people feel that they have diarrhoea if they pass several soft stools in a day, but strictly speaking it is the passage of fluid with no shape or solid mass.

Constipation

For some constipation is passing fewer, harder stools daily, for others it can mean less frequent movements with large stools. Normal frequency varies between individuals, from one motion daily to two weekly. A common feature to many IBS sufferers is small 'rabbit pellet' motions, which are the result of spasmodic bowel movements.

Irritability

This refers to the ease with which the system is 'upset', producing symptoms of pain, distension and flatulence. Some people attribute the upsets to certain foods.

Colitis and links with IBS

'Itis' means irritation or inflammation. This is redness, heat, swelling and pain. Colon is another name for the whole intestine. Colitis is a combination of the two words meaning inflammation of the intestinal wall. It is not a motility problem, although it may cause changes in patterns of movement. Its main feature is pain, which doesn't come and go, is often worse after food and could be accompanied by constipation or diarrhoea.

Inflammation can lead to ulceration as the mucus lining is eroded by the inflammatory process. This would then be called **ulcerative colitis**. Diarrhoea is a particular feature of ulcerative colitis, when the lining may be extensively ulcerated which prevents it from removing water and bicarbonate from the bowel contents. An irritable bowel could become inflamed, then you would be described as suffering from IBS *and* colitis. This is quite common, although there is no evidence that IBS is the cause of the inflammation.

Crohn's and coeliac disease

Crohn's disease

Crohn's disease is a condition of inflammation and ulceration in the small intestine, though sometimes it spreads a little way into the bowel. It is noted for causing weight loss, fatigue and diarrhoea. It interferes with the absorption of nutrients, so all sorts of deficiencies occur which cause anaemia, bone loss, skin problems etc. *It is not a form of IBS*. Some researchers think that immune problems in the digestive tract are linked to this disease, and it appears to run in families so there may be a genetic fault.

Coeliac disease

Coeliac disease is also called gluten enteropathy. It is a condition which is not very well understood and is quite separate from both IBS and colitis, as it has particular features and a specific cause. The symptoms are similar to Crohn's, but in coeliac disease the higher part of the GIT is damaged by a protein present in wheat and other grains. The essential absorptive lining 'withers' so problems arise due to deficiencies of vitamins, minerals, fats and even starch. Weight loss, skin problems and fatty diarrhoea are the main features.

There are some immune problems which are associated with this disease. The GIT appears to lack IgA, an immune cell which protects the GIT against infection. It isn't certain if this is an acquired defect or a hereditary one. Bottle fed babies appear to have far less IgA than breast fed babies. This is because breast milk contains IgA which gives a head start to the baby's own production. It is not known whether there is any connection between this early immune deficiency and later development of coeliac disease.

The changes which take place in the GIT can be seen on endoscopy, so there is no need for misdiagnosis. It is not an allergic condition and is massively over-diagnosed as 'wheat allergy' by patients and alternative practitioners. Removal of gluten cures Coeliac disease, so it will not be included in this book.

Patients and practitioners who suspect gluten enteropathy – coeliac disease – should refer to a hospital consultant for diagnostic tests. It does seem, however, that some people do better with less wheat products in their diet and the possible reasons for this will be discussed later.

Diverticulitis

This condition really belongs to the group of colitis diseases. Diverticuli are pouches in the sides of the bowel wall, formed (it is thought) by contraction of the muscles on a bowel which contains no bulking fibre. When these become inflamed, or infected by bacteria, fermentation distends them and causes pain. This can be quite severe. It is possible to see diverticuli on barium meal x-ray, so the diagnosis is quite specific, but the treatment is generally the same as for IBS so it is included in this book.

Causes of IBS

Irritable bowel syndrome is a group of symptoms which may have a number of causes, all occurring together. To understand this we have to take a wholistic view of all the factors which influence the digestive system.

What influences the digestion

- emotions
- lifestyle
- infections
- dysbiosis
- diet
- inherited tendencies
- exercise
- allergies
- drugs.

How do your emotions affect your digestion?

Anxiety is a type of fear, which is part of our primitive protective behaviour. It makes us alert and ready to respond to attack.

- Sympathetic nerve transmitters are mobilised. These

cause increased heart rate and constriction of visceral blood vessels (digestion), with greater blood flow to exercising somatic muscle (arms and legs).

- Digestive muscles first go through a phase of action (dumping their contents), then all secretory activity ceases (dry mouth).

It seems that some of these reactions can become chronic (long-lasting). A health writer called Hans Selye called this 'permanent stress adaptation'. This means that the digestive system is frequently under-secreting and under-perfused with blood. The muscles of the GIT don't move smoothly in rhythmic pulses but in spasmodic jerks as the regulation of nerve messages is uneven. This may also account for some cases of acid reflux (heartburn), where the movement of the sphincter is spasmodic. We may contribute to this uneven nerve stimulation by:

- 'binge stimulation' – lots of coffee to wake up
- and 'binge relaxation' – lots of alcohol to unwind.

Anger increases tension in muscles as sympathetic nerve transmission to them increases. This affects the digestive muscles as well, so the rhythmic movement of peristalsis is interrrupted. This can cause constipation, which is often accompanied by wind and gives an uncomfortable bloated feeling. If constipation becomes chronic, eventually diarrhoea may occur as the impacted faeces irritate the bowel and it produces spasmodic movements in reaction. This is often what gives rise to the alternating pattern of bowel movement which is so characteristic of IBS.

Emotional shocks can cause quite sudden constipation, which gradually resolves as the body and mind relax again over days or weeks.

Effects of lifestyle on digestion

- People who drive for a living, work long hours or shifts, often have uneven eating patterns which may contribute to variable bowel movements.
- Some people eat nothing in the early part of the day and present their digestive system with an enormous meal later. This also means that they have to rely on one meal for all their nutritional requirements.
- Missing the call to empty the bowel (defaecate) can cause the muscles to go into spasm, faeces become harder as water continues to be removed, dry stools are harder to pass and the muscles react even more spasmodically.
- Eating directly before brisk exercise causes muscular spasm, especially at the two bends (flexures) in the large intestine.This is what is known as a 'stitch' which you feel just below the ribcage on either side of your body.

Infections

Bacteria and their toxins can cause severe 'upset' to the bowel by irritating the inner surface. This causes increased movement and reduces absorption of water. The usual symptom of infection is diarrhoea and large spasms of muscles known as gripes, although fungal infections are more associated with wind and constipation. Candida albicans is a fungus which is often blamed for symptoms of IBS, but it is over-diagnosed – colonoscopic tests are required for firm diagnosis. Vaginal thrush does not necessarily indicate candidal overgrowth.

Dysbiosis

This means that the bowel does not have a normal content of digestive enzymes and 'friendly' bacteria which help to protect against infection. Sometimes the bowel fails to re-establish this normal balance after an infection, or after antibiotic treatment, and symptoms of wind, constipation or diarrhoea become chronic as food isn't digested properly and water is not removed.

Dietary causes

The food we eat and what we drink affect the way our digestion works.

Fibre is a part of vegetable and fruit which isn't absorbed by the body, but passes through the GIT giving 'bulk' for the walls to grip on for the rhythmic squeezing and propelling movements called peristalsis. Without fibrous bulk the walls constrict too much and bulges occur at weak points as mentioned before under diverticulitis.

Bulk is also important to start peristalsis – almost no movement occurs without sufficient bulk to initiate it. Bran was once considered the ideal fibre, as it swells up in the GIT giving pure bulk, but herbalists prefer fruit, vegetables and seeds as sources because they provide other nutrients, whereas bran provides none. It also contains a lot of phytic acid, which, if unmodified, interferes with vitamin and mineral absorption. Pure bran is now considered to be too filling for children, who need smaller amounts of food with more concentrated nutrients. In fact too much bran increases the dryness of faeces and causes wind, griping and constipation, the very symptoms that IBS sufferers dread.

Can some foods cause IBS?

Many people with IBS complain that several foods 'set them off'. For some people the list of foods they 'can't eat' is longer than those they can. True food allergies are quite rare, it is probably truer to say that an irritable bowel finds all food a little difficult and the more irritable it gets, the more foods cause problems. Raw fruit and vegetables top the list of problem foods, as these are the very foods which we need for vitamin health. This book will explain how to use herbs to soothe, heal and retrain the bowel so that it can accept these useful foods again.

How drinking water affects bowel movement

If you don't drink enough water your bowel contents may be too dry and reabsorption of water from the bowel makes it worse. Dry, hard stools are harder to pass so straining may cause the veins to bulge, causing piles.This is often accompanied by flatulence and bloating.

Do some people have an inherited tendency to IBS?

Most people experience some variation in bowel movements according to how much they eat and drink and how they feel.

It seems that some people have less tension in their gut muscles than others. They may have been told they have a 'lax bowel' and have suffered constipation since childhood. These people may have relied on laxatives, or had them supplied by mothers who were brought up to believe that 'once a day' was essential. The bowel may have become dependent on laxatives and require more stimulation than usual to obtain a movement, so the natural tendency is exacerbated.

The effect of exercise on your bowel

Muscle contractions in the abdominal muscles help to massage the large bowel and move contents along.

- Standing and gentle strolling allow the stomach and small intestine to process food more efficiently as working with gravity helps keep acid in its place and propel food downwards.

- Exercises in the morning before breakfast relax muscles and aid digestion.

Getting into a car, or sitting hunched at a desk directly after meals can cause cramped muscles and indigestion.

Can allergies cause IBS?

There doesn't seem to be any example of a true allergy causing digestive problems. Coeliac disease, as mentioned above, is a condition caused by defective enzymes, with possible immune deficiency association.

Milk intolerance is also due to lacking an enzyme (lactase) which splits milk starch (lactose). When lactose remains in the bowel it attracts water, causing very loose motions(osmotic diarrhoea). Removing milk from the diet resolves the problem.

Many people give up all wheat products, because they feel that it is responsible for all their digestive problems. It may be that they were eating too much refined starch (low fibre) or bran-rich bread which wasn't made with yeast – which breaks down phytic acid – or that their usual sandwich fillings were too salty. It may be possible that flour improvers are a digestive problem, or that the quantity of bread consumed left little room for more nutritious foods. One must keep an open mind and try eliminations one at a time for a limited period before reintroducing them.

Drugs

Nicotine in cigarettes causes small blood vessels to constrict, so it shuts off blood supply to the digestive system. Smoking cigarettes is associated with an extra risk for stomach ulcers and cancer. Most people have the urge to smoke directly after a meal just when they need their blood supply most! This affects absorption, especially of vitamins, and can cause griping. It may be a factor in the development of IBS and colitis.

Chemicals in coffee can be very irritant to the gut lining, these are not removed from decaffeinated varieties. Coffee helps to increase movement when taken after a meal, so can be seen as a beneficial digestive stimulant, but may be too much for a sensitive bowel.

2

What conventional medicine can offer

If you visit your doctor with symptoms of IBS and colitis he or she may arrange tests such as endoscopy to view the small intestine by camera, or barium meal which gives an x-ray view of the bowel, or proctoscopy to view the lower bowel by camera. You may be prescribed the following medicines which control the symptoms:

- Mobility Agents:
  - anti-spasmodics
  - muscle relaxants
  - opioid analgesics.
- Laxatives:
  - bowel stimulants
  - bulking agents
  - osmotic laxatives
  - faecal softeners.
- Anti-inflammatories:
  - steroids
  - aminosalicylates.

You may also be offered the following medicines to alter the emotional influences on your bowel:

- Tranquillisers.
- Anti-depressants:
  - MAOI's
  - tricyclics
  - SSRI's.
- Adsorbents.

Mobility agents

Anti-spasmodics

Main examples

- Merbentyl
- Kolanticon
- Buscopan.

These are usually the first choice for patients suffering from IBS symptoms, as it is thought mainly to be a disorder of motility (movement). They reduce the effect acetylcholine (the main nerve transmittor in the GIT) has on its target organs – fewer messages are received, so bowel movement and digestive secretions are greatly reduced. This can relieve pain and diarrhoea if spasm is the cause.

Problems with use

They reduce secretions everywhere, so tickly coughs may occur due to lack of bronchial secretions, lack of sweat may produce dry itchy skin, and nutrients may not be broken down due to reduced digestive enzymes. They may interfere with normal penile erection, as they interfere with muscles in blood vessels, preventing dilation and secretion of components of semen. All these ill-effects stop when you cease taking these medicines.

It is interesting to note that most of this group is derived from herbs – atropine from deadly nightshade and hyoscine from henbane.

Muscle relaxants

Main examples

- mebeverine (brand name Colofac, Fybogel) also contains mebeverine
- alverine (brand names Spasmonal, Avercol) also contains isphagula husk, a bulk laxative.

These work on smooth (visceral) muscle directly by changing the balance of calcium, potassium and sodium in the muscle fibre cells. This prevents muscles from remaining tense for longer than necessary for normal movement. This doesn't appear to cause any side-effects elsewhere in the body.

Problems with use

The medicinal effect lasts longer than the usual relaxation phase of a muscle movement, so people who don't have very good bowel muscle strength could find that they cause constipation. IBS sufferers often have reduced bowel muscle activity due to lack of fruit and vegetable fibre, which they find irritating.

Opioid analgesics

Main examples

- codeine (brand name Diarrest)
- loperamide (brand names Imodium, Diareze)
- co-phenotrope (brand name Lomotil) also contains atropine
- morphine (brand name Diocalm) also contains kaolin.

These derive their name from the fact that they are in the same chemical family as opium poppy extracts. They act on brain centres which send messages to visceral muscle to remain tense and stop moving. For this reason these medicines are also called anti-motility agents. They also act on heart and respiratory muscles and activate the vomiting reflex in sensitive individuals. They exacerbate digestive muscle tension caused by anxiety, as they use the same pathways, so that they are not meant to be used in cases of chronic diarrhoea which is really a spasmodic reaction to super-tension and constipation.

The brain develops more receptors for these chemicals

very quickly, so that you need more to achieve the same effect (tolerance) and the gut muscles respond less to your own nerve messages then need the drug to activate them (dependence). They are used to halt extreme loss of fluid and nutrients, usually in infections of the GIT such as dysentery which is expected to have a short duration.

Some researchers think that regular use of codeine-type medicines can cause increase in pain when withdrawn, because they inhibit the body's natural pain killers (endorphins).

Laxatives

These can be divided into three groups:

Bulking agents

Main examples

- isphagula husk (brand names Regulan, Fybogel) also contains mebeverine
- sterculia bean husk (brand name Normacol)
- methylcellulose (brand name Celevac)
- bran (brand name Trifyba) astonishingly marketed to the doctor at £3.28 for 175g, to the patient at prescription price. Currently sells for £6 per 25kg to retailers.

These work by swelling in the bowel, absorbing water and providing bulk which stimulates peristaltic muscle movement.

Problems with use

These can increase constipation where the GIT moves slowly or spasmodically. They frequently cause wind and bloating as bacterial fermentation is increased by indigestible fibre. Bran contains large amounts of phytic acid, which inhibits mineral and vitamin absorption. All bulk laxatives need to absorb water to swell sufficiently in the bowel, so large amounts of water must be drunk with them to avoid uncomfortable constipation.

Bowel stimulants

Bowel stimulants work by 'irritating' the lining of the bowel so that it moves more rapidly. They have different modes of action.

- Senna contains anthraquinones which are absorbed into the bloodstream and delivered to the bowel 8-10 hours later.
- Bisacodyl works both directly and via the bloodstream.

Problems with use

The bowel muscle becomes tolerant and dependant so the tendency to constipation increases. Anthraquinones can cause permanent damage to the bowel wall with long-term use.

Osmotic laxatives

These work by attracting water into the bowel. The main types are:

- Milk of Magnesia
- Andrews liver salts
- Epsom salts
- lactulose,(sold as Regulose) a milk sugar which can cause wind and bloating.

Faecal softeners

These can be:

- taken orally (liquid paraffin)
- or used in suppositories (glycerol).

Liquid paraffin acts as a lubricant, and is not digested in any way, but it interferes with vitamin and mineral absorption and can be absorbed into the bloodstream directly where it causes serious problems, especially in the lungs.

Anti-inflammatories

Steroids

These are prescribed where there is inflammation or ulcer, prominent in colitis and Crohn's disease.

Main examples

- prednisolone
- dexamethasone
- methylprednisolone
- hydrocortisone.

They prevent a key chemical from being made by white blood cells. This reduces the inflammatory cascade of chemicals from taking place, so swelling, pain and leakiness disappear.

Problems with use

Steroids are produced in the body naturally in small amounts in response to infections and injury. They are involved in making all soft tissue structures in the body, such as skin, muscle, GIT and blood vessel linings. When taken over long periods (six months or more) the synthetic steroids suppress these natural processes, as well as the production of adrenal hormones. This can result in muscle wasting, leaky capillaries, easy bruising, protein deficiency in bones, diabetes and succumbing to infections. Hydrocortisone also causes water retention as it affects potassium and sodium balance. Steroid drugs also affect mood – withdrawal can cause feelings of depression.

Aminosalicylates

Main examples

- sulphasalazine (brand name Salazopyrin)
- mesalazine (brand names Asacol, Pentasa).

These interfere with the growth and multiplication of bacteria. This action also inhibits the activity of enzymes which break down tissue in ulcer formation.

Problems with use

These medicines also inhibit blood cell formation, and they frequently cause irritation and damage to kidneys and liver because they form crystal deposits and interfere with enzyme systems.

Tranquillisers

These are also known as anxiolytics. They have been largely replaced by the modern anti-depressants, as they are now thought to be too sedative for daily use and they create dependence. They are prescribed to alleviate the feelings of anxiety which can cause motility problems in the digestive system.

Main examples

- benzodiazepines (brand names Diazepam, Lorazepam, Temazepam)
- valium.

Tranquillisers act on the brain, especially the limbic system, a group of cells which plays an important role in mood creation (feelings of general well-being). The number of messages sent to visceral and skeletal muscle is reduced, so less tension is maintained. Calmer, slower movement of bowel muscle may result.

Problems with use

These medicines interfere with fine muscle movements, so one may become clumsy and they affect the ability to think clearly, as well as remember recent items and events. When used at night they often have a 'hangover' effect in the morning which makes it difficult to feel fully awake.

Anti-depressants

These are prescribed to alleviate feelings of anxiety, which are often linked to depression. They have largely replaced the tranquillisers (mentioned above). Many patients feel wrongly diagnosed if they are given anti-depressants, but they are used for their relaxing effects, which are less sedative than the earlier anxiolytics. The mood elevating effect may be seen as secondary in many cases. There are three main types.

MAOIs (monoamine oxidase inhibitors)

Main examples

- phenelzine (brand name Nardil)

- isocarboxazid
- moclobemide (brand name Manerix).

These preserve neurotransmittors such as noradrenaline, which helps to maintain an elevated, alert state of mind and a sense of energy (part of the fight or flight reaction). They react with fermented products – cheese, soya and yeast extract, pickles and some beans. They aren't used for mild anxiety now as they are really best suited to certain types of severe depression (marked by lethargy and torpor).

Tricyclics

Main examples

- amitryptilene (brand names Lentizol, Tryptizol)
- clomipramine (brand name Anafranil)
- imipramine (brand name Tofranil)
- dothiepin (brand name Prothiaden).

These preserve supplies of noradrenaline and hydroxytyramine (nerve transmitters in the brain). These keep the brain alert as well as producing a feeling of well-being. (In hibernating animals these chemicals are reduced.)

Problems with use

It is known that certain phases of the sleep cycle are suppressed, especially that known as REM (rapid eye movement) sleep. It isn't known exactly how important this type of sleep is and long term use of these drugs can prevent satisfactory sleeping patterns from being established. Some researchers think that the brain becomes dependent on these medicines as many patients report intractable depression occurring on every attempt to reduce dosage or stop taking them.

SSRIs (selective serotonin re-uptake inhibitors)

This is the new generation of 'stress busters'. The group includes:

- paroxetine (brand name Seroxat)
- fluoxetine (brand name Prozac)
- sertraline (brand name Lustral).

They preserve supplies of serotonin, a neuro-transmittor in the brain which maintains a buoyant mood and wakefulness.

Problems with use

Initially (for two to three weeks) insomnia, anorexia, headache and nausea occur. These problems subside as a sense of well-being continues to increase over several months. This may change into a mild sense of euphoria, which distances you slightly from true social awareness, so people on these medicines may find they are able to be a little too bold, rude or even uncaring (even about themselves). Some people lose their sense of self-preservation (which is based on anxiety). Where this coincides with an unresolved depression, people can make serious errors of judgement. Stopping doesn't seem to cause withdrawal but there is usually a 'trough' of irritable depression a couple of weeks after ceasing medication, which lifts in about the same time.

Adsorbents

These are usually mineral clays such as kaolin, which hold water and adhere to the gut wall for some time. This slows the action of the bowels. They interfere with mineral absorption from the gut and should not be used for long periods.

3

Using herbs to treat IBS and Colitis

Herbal medicine is the leading alternative to conventional pharmaceutical treatment. When herbalists make up a prescription for patients with bowel problems, they take into account all the factors which contribute to their health and try to improve all the systems which are affected by digestive deficiencies. This is called a wholistic approach. It is the main difference between conventional and herbal treatment. In addition to prescribing herbal medicine, herbalists would want a patient to start exercises and dietary changes in a strategy to maintain general well-being.

Aims of herbal treatment

- Reduce inflammation and infection
- Relieve pain
- Relax muscles and improve regular movement
- Reduce nervous tension
- Improve blood supply
- Increase nutrient digestion and absorption.

The patient would be prescribed some of the following

anti-infective herbs which reduce the bacterial population of the bowel, which is sometime an effect of IBS and a cause of colitis.

- **Anti-spasmodic** and **muscle relaxant herbs** which are used to create easy, regular movement of the bowel wall.
- **Nervine relaxants** which are taken to reduce the impact of psychological tension on the digestive system.
- **Circulatory tonics** which enable the huge capillary network to feed the wall of the bowel and carry away nutrients to their target organs.
- **Digestive stimulants** which increase secretion and so improve the breakdown and absorption of nutrients, which enhances overall energy and health.

How herbs work

Herbs contain small quantities of chemicals, compared to modern pharmaceutical products which extract or synthesise one chemical in much larger amounts. This means there is no danger of sudden physiological changes which cause side-effects. For example, valerian appears to improve the quality of your sleep as well as helping you to doze off and doesn't cause a sluggish feeling in the morning, because the chemicals it contains are in very small amounts and don't last long in the body. This lower level of activity may be disappointing if you want to be 'knocked out' but using herbs like valerian as part of a plan to restore sleep patterns can be an effective alternative to stronger, single chemicals like the well-known sedative, valium (derived originally from valerian).

Most herbs contain a large number of active constituents which work together to create one or more effects. The more we find out about herbs, the more we realise that each constituent is a valued part of the whole, negative effects balanced by positive ones. A good example follows.

Recently much has been made of a research trial which showed that a St John's Wort preparation made liver enzymes more active, which reduced the effect of other drugs taken at the same time because they were metabolised before reaching their target. The St John's Wort preparation used was standardised to contain a larger amount of one constituent – hypericin, than all the others. Not only has hypericin failed to show anti-depressant activity on its own in repeated trials, but another ingredient – hyperforin – has been shown to counterbalance hypericin in its effect on liver enzymes. Many other research trials on St John's Wort have shown no adverse effect on other drugs and doctors in Germany continue to prescribe it as a favoured anti-depressant. Similar bad publicity surrounds liquorice, where glycyrrhizin is thought to raise blood pressure, but in fact dozens of other constituents act to lower it, in particular by diuresis (elimination of water).

There are many more examples of this sort of balanced action. Where two or more constituents act together to create the same effect this is known as synergy. These are particular features of herbal medicine which enable it to support the wholistic approach very well.

How long do herbs take to work?

Although some herbs act swiftly, like the relaxant valerian, herbal remedies generally act slowly and their effect is cumulative. They gently rebalance physiological processes, as though switch after switch is thrown until the full effect is achieved. This can take weeks, sometimes months, but it is worth waiting for, as the risk of side-effects is very low due to the tiny amounts of chemicals involved.

How do herbal remedies get to their target?

Herbal compounds need to be absorbed across the wall of the digestive tract, so they have to be released from their structures (stem, root, leaf, flower or berry etc) first of all. Hot water and alcohol do some of this job for us, so that teas and tinctures are more easily absorbed than tablets and capsules, which need to be broken down physically before the active chemicals are separated from the inert matter to which they are attached. All food and medicine passes through the liver (in the blood circulation) before it finally enters the body tissues, where it is used.

Sometimes chemical compounds need help in crossing through the wall of the digestive tract into the blood stream. Carrier chemicals can be attached to compounds and ferry them through channels in the gut lining. Hydrochloride is frequently found to be part of conventional drug names as it has this function.

Herbal compounds often have an advantage over synthesised chemicals in this respect, as they have naturally occurring carrier chemicals already attached to them. This is what is meant by affinity. Herbs are said to have a greater affinity for the human body, like spare parts, dedicated to a particular engine made by the same manufacturer.

Are herbs safe?

All the herbs which British Herbalists use are safe when used in the correct dose for the right ailment. The herbs mentioned in this book have been selected for their safety in untrained hands, although you may need professional help with your diagnosis. The National Institute of Medical Herbalists (NIMH – see page 140) maintains an extensive data bank and works with government watchbodies to ensure safety of its herbs. Recently some attention was given to the group of compounds called pyrrolizidine alkaloids, present in several plants including comfrey, because they can cause (reversible) damage to the liver if ingested in large quantities. The evidence on comfrey is not based on human case studies and the research involved feeding rats exclusively on large amounts of comfrey. There is only one reported case of human toxicity world-wide, which concerned a woman who took comfrey tea many times a day concurrently with illegal drugs in high doses over a long period. Several governments, including that of Britain, made moves to ban its use. After extensive discussions with the NIMH, it was agreed to limit use to the guidelines given above, and restrict the root (which contains more P.A.'s) to external use only. In this way herbalists acknowledge the potential risk and demonstrate the history of safe use.

Combining herbs with orthodox medication

Some drugs are altered by liver enzymes, so that they enter the main blood circulation in a different form. Some herbs (especially **bitters**) stimulate the liver cells to work harder, or cause more liver cells to be active and this can affect other drugs because the liver removes them from circulation before they have had a chance to do their work. Digoxin is one of these and is also a drug with a 'narrow therapeutic window'. This means that the difference between an insufficient, a beneficial and a harmful dose is very small, so that small changes in the amount getting through to the bloodstream may result in the drug not working as it should. Two other drugs like this are Cyclosporin, used to prevent transplant rejection, and Phenytoin, an anti-epileptic. It is very important to check with a qualified herbalist and let your doctor know if you are adding herbal medicine to medication you are currently using.

There are many herbs which can be taken safely with other medicines, so don't feel deterred from trying, but do seek professional advice. Herbs can be used to offset the side-effects of necessary medication, like indigestion or nausea. They may enable you to take less of a remedy which you need, but which has troublesome side-effects. The important thing is how you feel, and that you don't endanger your health. It may be simple to ask your doctor to monitor blood levels of drugs and adjust the dose if necessary.

It would not be wise to embark on herbal medicine without medical supervision if you are on anti-psychotic medication, as you may not be aware that your mental condition has deteriorated when your current medication ceases to work. You may have strong feelings about the disadvantages of your drugs, but may not realise how your behaviour is changing and affecting others badly. It is possible to have herbal medicine for other complaints while on medication for psychosis, but you must consult your doctor first and allow yourself to be monitored.

If you are on chemotherapy for cancer, it would be better to wait until your treatment has finished before taking herbal medicine, unless you are looking for help with troublesome side effects such as nausea or diarrhoea. Several herbs can help here without reducing the effectiveness of your anti-cancer drugs.

Drugs to be careful with	Conditions to be careful with
Digoxin	Pregnancy
Phenytoin	Epilepsy
Anti-psychotics	Schizophrenia, psychosis
Immune suppressants	Organ transplants
Anti-cancer drugs	Allergies

Sometimes over the counter herbal medicines are labelled with contra-indications. This is required by law in Germany. It means for example that you will be told if you shouldn't take the medicine if you are pregnant, taking another specific medication, have an allergy or a certain medical condition. This will become more common in Europe in the future.

The advantages of using whole plant preparations

Herbalists insist on using whole, unaltered products to guarantee the sort of benefits we claim for them. We believe that plants would only have gained a historical reputation for certain effects if their constituents were robust enough to maintain the same effect wherever they were grown or whatever minor differences there might be between local plant populations. If only one variety in one particular year made someone feel better, its reputation would not have stood the test of time.

The current trend, based on scientific research, is to standardise the process of growing, harvesting and storing herbs, so that their use is sustainable and patients get the best value from them. Medical herbalists also recommend using whole, unaltered preparations, as nature presented them, so that each constituent is represented in its natural amounts. This is the type of preparation on which traditional knowledge is based. It is also useful to remember that patients vary much more than plants do!

The affinity of herbs

Many herbs show a greater affinity for the human body than synthetic medicines. This is because they have compounds and molecules attached which make them more easily absorbed into body cells and tissues. These are often in the sugar family. Some are known as glycosides and these and their relatives, monosaccharides, are attracting a lot of interest in the modern research world. These carrier chemicals enable herbal compounds to enter target cells more easily, and may explain how herbs can have an effect, even at quite low doses.

The constituents of herbs

Another advantage of herbal medicine is that there are so many different plants with similar actions, but different combinations of constituents. You can change from one to the other to avoid becoming tolerant or developing sensitivities. For example, there are many anti-inflammatory herbs, each with its own supplementary actions including hormonal, diuretic, anti-spasmodic and relaxing effects. Herbs may act on several different aspects of a condition at the same time, like garlic which provides help for our circulation on several levels. As an antibiotic it repairs the damage caused by wear and tear on the insides of our blood vessels. As a digestive stimulant it helps the absorption of sugars and fats from the bloodstream. As a circulatory tonic it reduces the stickiness of platelets, dilates the capillaries, causes mild sweating and increases kidney activity, so it helps to protect against strokes and lowers blood pressure slightly.

Herbal applications

Herbal remedies include conventional applications such as:

- anti-inflammatories
- laxatives
- iron tonics
- anti-spasmodics.

You can also find herbs whose actions are not found in conventional drug descriptions. Mostly this is because of their complexity, which is best reflected in the older names for their applications. We can include here:

- relaxants
- carminatives
- astringents
- anti-infectives
- demulcents
- circulatory tonics
- digestive tonics (relaxing or stimulating).

Anti-inflammatories

Inflammation causes pain and damage if unchecked. Anti-inflammatories work by intervening in the inflammatory process at different levels. Some act by reducing the number of immune cells produced in response to injury, for example chamomile reduces the number of mast cells which are part of the swelling process. Some herbs stabilise cell membranes so they don't break down or allow excess secretion. This may be done by inhibiting chemicals such as bradykinin, serotonin and histamine, which also make small blood vesssels leak fluid. It is thought that mucus membrane tonics such as elderflower work in this way.

Laxatives

There are several different sorts of laxative

- bulky
- stimulant
- relaxing
- bitter.

Bulky laxatives

These add solid mass to the contents of the bowel. This stimulates the regular movement called peristalsis, which is ongoing but increases when messages from bowel wall nerve endings are relayed via the lower brain stem (an unconscious area of the brain).

Stimulant laxatives

These work by irritating the bowel wall which increases its movement rapidly. They generally are not direct, but absorbed into the bloodstream first and delivered some time (8-10 hours) later. These are not gentle laxatives. If they cause excessive muscular movement it is known as griping. They are always taken with carminatives to ensure a calm action.

Relaxing laxatives

Generally these are the same herbs as in the nervine and muscle relaxing category. They work directly on muscle to relieve tension.

Bitter laxatives

These increase the bile acid content of the bowel, so soften its contents and stimulate peristalsis by reflex.

Iron tonics

These provide iron to replace supplies lost with persistent bleeding. Herbs such as parsley and watercress also contain Vitamin C, which enhances the absorption of iron, so they are a very good source of this mineral.

Anti-spasmodics

These herbs reduce muscle contraction or allow it to relax again. There are two sorts: central acting herbs, which reduce brain activity so fewer stimulating messages are sent to muscles, and peripherally acting herbs which act directly on the muscle fibre cells. These don't reduce messages sent by the brain, so there is rarely a sedative effect.

Relaxants

Muscle relaxants

These usually work directly on the muscle, preventing it from contracting so it is maintained in a relaxed state. This is a stronger effect than an anti-spasmodic, the muscles may feel a little flaccid. Where this action occurs in the smooth muscle of the bowel, peristalsis may be halted. Some muscle relaxants act on somatic muscle as well and may be interfering with reception of messages from the brain. The actions of muscle relaxants and anti-spasmodics are very close and some writers do not distinguish between them.

Nervine relaxants

Herbal nervine relaxants relieve mental tension and restore nervous activity to a normal level, whereas sedatives reduce brain activity to below normal functioning level. This can improve concentration rather than impairing it, so it is a good example of a balancing action for which herbs are well known. These herbs work in two ways: some act centrally, by reducing the brain's sensitivity to nerve messages from the periphery (skin, joints, muscles etc); others act on nerve centres in the spinal cord or on nerve endings in the skin, reducing the number of messages sent from the periphery to the brain. Nervine relaxants tend to act centrally, muscle relaxants act peripherally, many herbs do both at once.

Carminatives

These usually contain constituents which are antiseptic and anti-spasmodic. They relieve muscular spasm and dispel wind by reducing bacterial fermentation in the bowel which produces gases and acting directly on smooth muscle to relax it. They are extremely important in treating bowel disorders.

Astringents

These reduce the secretions of cells or reduce leakiness so surfaces may become less swollen, or less 'hyperactive', perhaps feeling 'drier'. Mucus membrane tonics work in this way, reducing catarrhal secretions and swelling in sinus linings. This is also a useful action in herbal treatment of IBS, where GIT linings are swollen, leaky (allowing large, allergenic proteins through), over-producing mucus or allowing water to leak back from surrounding tissues. Many herbs which contain tannins are astringent in a different way – they coagulate protein, so seal raw surfaces and prevent leakiness. This astringency can also contribute to the anti-infective effect (see below) as tannins coagulate bacterial protein thus killing them. Tannin-rich astringents relieve diarrhoea by coating the gut linings and numbing them.

Anti-infectives

These have a stronger anti-bacterial action than carminatives. They sometimes contain volatile oils and sometimes pungent (hot-tasting) compounds which stimulate digestive secretion by irritating GIT surfaces. For this reason they are often avoided in cases of ulceration.

These herbs have several modes of action. They reduce bacterial population by coagulation (astringents), irritation (spices) and interfering with life processes of bacterial cells (sulphur compounds).

Demulcents

Demulcent herbs soothe the surfaces they pass over, reducing messages of pain and irritation by direct action. They generally contain mucilage, a starchy substance which is not absorbed like calorific starches, so they last into the lower bowel where they often form a temporary protective surface which reduces heat, pain and inflammation. Sometimes they are known as emollients. Herbs which combine astringent with demulcent effects are often known as healers. 'Vulneraries' have these qualities and antiseptic ones as well.

Circulatory tonics

These relax and dilate blood vessels, which lowers pressure. They increase blood flow to all parts of the body including internal organs such as the bowel wall. They lower cholesterol, improve the elasticity of blood vessels and make them less fragile as well as reducing clotting or platelet aggregation, so helping to prevent thrombosis. Menopausal women often avoid using the herbs which stimulate blood flow (such as chilli, ginger, mustard and horseradish) because they also increase sweating, which can be intolerable for women who experience severe hot flushes. Iron rich herbs may be considered as circulatory tonics as they provide the essential nutrition of the bowel wall itself and increase delivery of oxygen to other parts of the body. Peripheral circulatory tonics act on nerve endings in blood vessel walls. Central circulatory tonics work on the heart to improve performance or stabilise rhythm.

Digestive tonics

Stimulant tonics

- Increase digestive enzymes
- Increase protective linings
- Increase breakdown of foods

- Increase absorption of nutrients
- Increase bowel movement
- Increase elimination of waste.

Stimulant digestive tonics can be used to increase the secretion of the digestive organs by stimulating enzyme action in the liver as mentioned before, or by increasing the production and flow of bile (the bitters are noted for this action). Spices such as cayenne, ginger, horseradish and mustard act by irritating the secretory linings of the stomach and intestines, causing increase in all sorts of secretions including mucin, which protects the stomach from acid. These spices also cause dilation of blood vessels serving the gut wall, which helps to increase the absorption of nutrients. It is thought that pancreatic hormones may also be produced in response to some of these digestive herbs, so sugar, fat and protein digestion may be enhanced. This is the action we call digestive stimulation. It may increase the absorption and metabolism (breakdown and use) of the nutrients needed for general health.

Relaxing bitter tonics

These tonics are unique to herbal medicine. Nearly every country has a national favourite, the French drink gentian wine, Italians prefer vermouth, Mexicans use angostura and the British put their bitters in stouts and beers. You can still buy a formula known as Swedish bitters from pharmacies. Aromatic bitter herbs are also found in cookery traditions all over the world. In Britain sage, rosemary and thyme are used to improve the digestibility of meat and bean dishes.

How bitter tonics work

- Taste buds detect bitters.
- Nerve messages are sent to the brain.
- Reflex messages are sent to organs.
- Liver, pancreas and salivary glands are stimulated.
- Better absorption and elimination results.

Bitter taste buds are located at the back of your tongue. They are designed to detect poisons and trigger a gag reflex, so you spit out food which is bad for you. Humans can overcome the bitter revulsion reflex by three methods: telling ourselves it's good for us, adding nice flavours or adding alcohol! The body, however, still working to the primeval instruction handbook, initiates a process to rid the body of unwanted chemicals. The liver produces more enzymes and bile in response to messages sent in the brain from the tastebuds. Saliva flows abundantly to cleanse the mouth, activity in the stomach and pancreas increases, resulting in better absorption of nutrients and elimination of toxins. Distension, wind and bloating are relieved by bitter remedies. Pre-dinner drinks are good for you after all!

It is clear that herbs are similar in action to modern

chemical drugs (which are, after all, mostly designed on herbal models) but plants are complex and the chemicals they contain are in much smaller quantities, so they are often used differently. Persistence is usually more important than quantity – a little every day will slowly bring about change in physiological conditions. The combined advantages of synergy, low dosage, multi-level action, high affinity and low incidence of side effects have ensured that they will continue to be used as well as modern drugs in treatment of all kinds of disease.

4

Directory of useful herbs

You will need to use a number of strategies to relieve irritable bowel and colitis. Preventive approaches are covered in Chapter 6 on eating for healthy digestion. You can use the information in this section to select the right herbs. The case histories in Chapter 7 guide you in building classic recipes or tailoring one to your own individual needs.

Herbs are usually categorised by their actions, and each herb will have some primary and some secondary actions. In some the actions are of equal importance. To treat irritable bowel and colitis you may need anti-inflammatories, astringents laxatives, iron tonics, anti-spasmodics, relaxants, carminatives, anti-infectives, demulcents and digestive tonics. When you read the case histories later, you will see how this directory can be used to pick herbs from the various categories.

ANTI-INFLAMMATORIES

Chamomile	Fennel	Marigold	
Comfrey	Liquorice	Meadowsweet	Wild yam

Chamomile

Latin name	Matricaria recutita
Origin	Europe
Part used	Flower (This plant has been re-named several times recently, so you must specify small, cone-headed flowers with a single row of petals, which hang downwards. When you cut the flower head open it is hollow. This is currently known as German chamomile, but older lists still call it Roman chamomile, Anthemis nobilis).
Dose	1 teaspoon per cup Tincture 5ml, 1-3 times daily
Constituents	Volatile oil, flavonoids, coumarins, valerianic acid, sesquiterpene bitters, salicylates, tannins
Primary action	Relaxant
Secondary action	Anti-spasmodic Digestive tonic
How it works	Chamomile is one of the most complex herbs in common use. It has a little of almost every action shown by plants. The volatile oil is a central relaxant,it is also mildly antiseptic, and anti-inflammatory and carminative. Flavonoids are mildly diuretic, coumarins are anti-spasmodic, acting directly

	on smooth muscle. Sesquiterpene bitters are tonic to the liver and stimulate digestion, and bitter glycosides add to this action. Anti-inflammatory, pain relieving salicylates are present in small quantities, tannins are astringent to the wall of the bowel so alleviate diarrhoea.
Growing guide	Grows easily sown directly in pots or in a warm spot, but annual re-seeding is necessary as it 'won't stay put'.

Comfrey

Latin name	Symphytum officinalis
Origin	Europe
Part used	Leaf
Dose	1 teaspoon per cup Tincture 4ml 1-3 times daily, maximum 8 weeks
Constituents	Tannins, mucilage, allantoin, consolidine, phenols, pyrrolizidine alkaloids, Vitamin B^{12} , inulin, protein.
Primary action	Healing
Secondary action	Astringent Demulcent
How it works	Allantoin stimulates the formation of connective tissue, so promotes ulcer healing in the GIT. Its mucilage is demulcent, tannins are astringent and antibacterial. Phenols are antibacterial and some are anti-inflammatory.

Caution	Because of recent British government action, due to worries about pyrrolizidine alkaloids, you should not exceed the dose stated above, and make sure you obtain the correct variety as the P.A. content varies. Safe traditional use is based on Symphytum officinalis, selected here. (See page 46 for more detail.)
Growing guide	From piece of root. Tolerates poor and clay soil, can be invasive.

Fennel

Latin name	Foeniculum vulgaris
Origin	Europe
Part used	Seed
Dose	1 teaspoon per cup Tincture 4ml, 1-3 times daily
Constituents	Volatile oil, flavonoids, coumarins, sterols
Primary action	Carminative
Secondary action	Anti-inflammatory Diuretic
How it works	The volatile oil in fennel is strongly carminative reducing wind and bacterial fermentation. The flavonoids help to strengthen blood vessel walls, which reduces inflammatory leakiness. They are also responsible for the diuretic action (increasing elimination of water) which helps to remove water from the bowel and reduces diarrhoea. The coumarins are directly anti-spasmodic. The sterols don't contribute to the alleviation

	of bowel problems, but are weakly oestrogenic, so fennel may be the herb of choice for a menopausal woman with IBS.
Growing guide	Grows well in British gardens, but doesn't set seed as it prefers Mediterranean sun (don't blame it!).

Liquorice

Latin name	Glycyrrhiza glabra
Origin	Europe, Asia
Part used	Rhizome
Dose	1 teaspoon per cup Tincture 4ml, 1-3 times daily
Constituents	Glycosides, flavonoids, bitters, volatile oil, sterols, asparagin, coumarin, tannins, saponins, polysaccharides
Primary action	Anti-inflammatory Demulcent Healing
Secondary action	Adrenal tonic Expectorant Anti-spasmodic
How it works	The glycosides are tremendously sweet in taste (50 times sweeter than sugar) and have a number of important effects. They are anti-inflammatory (reducing histamine and acting on the early stages of the inflammatory process). They are anti-spasmodic and help to increase thin mucus production, so very useful for tickly coughs. They also inhibit

bacterial growth and have a cortisone-like action in improving repair mechanisms after injury or inflammation. They are central relaxants, with an anti-depressant mode of action. Both the coumarins and the volatile oil are anti-spasmodic, acting directly on smooth muscle in the bowel wall. The polysaccharides stimulate the production of immune cells such as interferon,the bitters are tonic to the liver and improve digestion. Flavonoids are diuretic so they offset the tendency for liquorice to make the body retain sodium.

Caution Large doses (more than three cups a day) for more than six weeks should be avoided, as there is a very small risk of raising blood pressure with some liquorice preparations. Liquorice sweets eaten in excess are noted for inducing raised blood pressure in some people.

Growing guide Can be grown in Britain, needs heat in summer and damp sandy soil, may turn woody in very cold winters, quite invasive.

Marigold

Latin name Calendula officinalis
Origin Europe
Part used Flower
Dose 1 teaspoon per cup
Tincture 4ml 1-3 times daily

Primary action	Healing Astringent
Secondary action	Anti-septic Anti-inflammatory
Constituents	Saponins, bitters, sterols, flavonoids, mucilage, chlorogenic acid
How it works	It is probable that the chlorogenic acid acts as a gentle antiseptic astringent, which together with the mucilage reduces inflammation in the bowel. Marigold is mildly bitter, so it is a gentle tonic to digestion. Flavonoids reduce permeability of capillaries, so it helps to reduce inflammation, especially in allergy. The saponins may help to reduce bacterial population. Sterols are possibly involved in the anti-inflammatory effects.
Growing guide	Sow seed directly into sunny spot in garden in early spring. Can be grown well in pots.

Meadowsweet

Latin name	Filipendula ulmaria
Origin	Europe
Part used	Leaf
Dose	1 teaspoon per cup Tincture 4ml, 1-3 times daily
Constituents	Volatile oil, salicylates, coumarins, tannins, phenols, flavonoids
Primary actions	Healing Anti-spasmodic

Secondary actions	Astringent Anti-inflammatory
How it works	The salicylates are pain relieving both in cases of ulcer and inflammation. They inhibit prostaglandins which carry messages about pain, fever and inflammation. Although salicylates are the chemicals associated with aspirin, which makes ulcers worse, meadowsweet is safe to use in inflamed gastric mucosa (stomach linings) because the salicylates are not converted into their active form until they have passed through the GIT lining into the bloodstream. The phenols and tannins are anti-septic and anti-inflammatory, so help to relieve ulceration on the GIT wall. The coumarins are muscle-relaxing and anti-spasmodic, acting directly on the bowel muscle. Flavonoids help to reduce permeability of small blood vessels, so reduce inflammatory fluid leakage.
Growing guide	Likes damp soil, will tolerate semi-shade, 6ft-tall white spires of flowers, suitable for back of borders.

Wild yam

Latin name	Dioscorea villosa
Origin	America
Part used	Root
Dose	1 teaspoon per cup Tincture 4ml, 1-3 times daily

Constituents	Steroids, saponins, alkaloids, tannins
Primary actions	Anti-spasmodic Anti-inflammatory
Secondary actions	Muscle relaxant Hormone agent
How it works	The anti-inflammatory, anti-spasmodic and muscle relaxant actions of wild yam are well known but not understood. It is a major source of hormone precursors for the human body. Its tannins have a mildly astringent effect on the bowel linings. It has become known recently as a herb for menopausal women but may be taken safely by men for spasmodic bowel conditions without side-effects (in fact this use pre-dates the hormonal discoveries).
Growing guide	Not suitable for British climate, it is a winding creeper, needing heat.

ASTRINGENTS

Agrimony	Bayberry	Cranesbill
Avens	Bistort	Tormentil

Agrimony

Latin name	Agrimonia eupatoria
Origin	Europe
Part used	Leaf
Dose	1 teaspoon per cup

	Tincture 4ml, 1-3 times daily
Primary actions	Astringent
	Bitter tonic
Secondary actions	Anti-viral
Constituents	Volatile oil, tannins, bitters, flavonoids, polysaccharides, coumarins
How it works	Agrimony is mildly bitter, so acts as a liver and digestive tonic. The tannins are responsible for the astringent action on the bowel wall. Coumarins are anti-spasmodic, working directly on smooth muscle. Poly saccharides are immune stimulant which may account for its reputation as an anti-viral. Flavonoids stabilise capillary membranes, reducing inflammation (this is a long-term action).
Growing guide	Sow directly, prefers dry sunny soil, will tolerate position next to hedge or wall.

Avens

Latin name	Geum urbanum
Origin	Europe
Part used	Leaf
Dose	1 teaspoon per cup
	Tincture 4ml, 1-3 times daily
Constituents	Phenols, bitter lactones, tannins
Primary actions	Astringent
	Bitter tonic
Secondary actions	Anti-inflammatory
How it works	Tannins are astringent and anti-inflammatory

by direct action on the bowel wall. Phenols are antibacterial, bitters promote better digestion and liver action.The net effect is a reduction of distension, wind, bloating, pain and diarrhoea.

Bayberry

Latin name	Myrica cerifera
Origin	America
Part used	Root
Dose	1 teaspoon per cup Tincture 2ml, 1-3 times daily
Constituents	Tannins, phenols, volatile oil, flavonoids
Primary actions	Astringent
Secondary actions	Circulatory stimulant
How it works	The tannins and phenols are astringent, anti-inflammatory and antibacterial. It is not known which constituents cause dilation of the capillaries, but bayberry is used for this effect to relieve feverish colds and lowers blood pressure slightly. It is used in mucus colitis and severe ulceration. It has a traditional use in cancers of the stomach and bowel.
Growing guide	8ft shrub, grows in swampy ground. Not tried in Britain.

Bistort

Latin name	Polygonum bistorta
Origin	Europe

Part used	Root
Dose	1/2 teaspoon per cup Tincture 2ml, 1-3 times daily
Constituents	Phenols, tannins, oxalic acid, flavonoids, mucilage
Primary actions	Astringent
Secondary actions	Demulcent
How it works	Bistort is mainly used as an anti-diarrhoeal, due to its astringent tannins and anti-bacterial phenols. Its astringent quality is also used to halt internal bleeding. It contains a small amount of mucilage which is demulcent in effect and offsets the mildy irritating effect of oxalic acid. This is another herb which has traditional use in cancers of the digestive system.
Growing guide	Grows wild in Britain, rather invasive.

Cranesbill

Latin name	Geranium maculatum
Origin	Europe
Part used	Root
Dose	1 teaspoon per cup Tincture 4ml, 1-3 times daily
Constituents	Tannins, pectin, gum
Primary actions	Astringent
Secondary actions	Anti-inflammatory
How it works	This herb has a fairly simple action, its tannins are astringent, they reduce bacteria and aid healing in inflamed tissues. It relieves

chronic diarrhoea and bleeding. Gum helps the healing process by soothing the GIT linings.

Growing guide Seeds itself readily, very hardy, prefers sunny areas.

Tormentil

Latin name Potentilla tormentilla
Origin Europe
Part used Root
Dose 1 teaspoon per cup
Tincture 4ml, 1-3 times daily
Constituents Tannins, bitters, gum
Primary actions Astringent
Secondary actions Tonic
How it works Tormentil has a large percentage of tannins, which are astringent and antibacterial. It is mildly bitter, so increases digestive activity. The gums contribute to the antibacterial effect and are slightly soothing to inflamed surfaces. It was traditionally used for bacterial GIT infections, such as dysentery, but can be used for chronic diarrhoea. Its astringent effect is very useful for relieving haemorrhoids, when it is used topically as a lotion or cream.
Growing guide Grows wild in Britain, rather invasive.

LAXATIVES

Alder buckthorn	Linseed	Senna
Butternut	Psyllium seed	Yellow dock
Cascara	Rhubarb	

Note: relaxing bitter tonics are also mildly laxative, and are covered in their relevant sections, see hops, lemon balm, vervein, and wormwood.

STIMULANT LAXATIVES

The stimulant laxatives (except butternut) all contain a group of chemicals called anthraquinone glycosides. These are substances which are absorbed in the upper part of the GIT and re-exported in the blood stream to the bowel, where they cause irritation to the wall. This causes rapid muscle movement in response, which can cause griping. Rhubarb and yellow dock are much milder in effect and don't cause griping. Yellow dock has the additional benefit of containing lots of iron. The others should always be taken with a carminative herb (see page 91).

Alder buckthorn

Latin name	Rhamnus frangula (also called frangula bark)
Origin	Europe
Part used	Berries
Dose	1 teaspoon per cup, taken once daily at night

Butternut

Latin name	Juglans cinararia

Origin	America
Part used	Inner bark
Dose	1 teaspoon per cup Tincture 4ml, 1-3 times daily
Constituents	Napthaquinones, tannins, volatile oil
Primary actions	Laxative
Secondary actions	Anti-microbial Bitter tonic
How it works	Butternut is a stimulant laxative which doesn't contain anthraquinones, but the bitter napthaquinone which is related but without griping effect. Bitters stimulate liver digestive activity, tannins are antibacterial and astringent, they contribute to the anti-microbial effect of the napthaquinones. The laxative effect is due to the napthaquinones. It is a safe tonic laxative, especially suitable for elderly people. It was formerly used to expel worms.
Growing guide	Large tree, not suitable for domestic gardens.

Cascara

Latin name	Rhamnus purshiana
Origin	West Indies
Part used	Bark

Rhubarb

Latin name	Rheum palmatum
Origin	China
Part used	Root

Senna

Latin name	Cassia senna
Origin	Africa
Part used	Seed pods
Dose	1 teaspoon per cup, taken once daily at night

Yellow Dock

Latin name	Rumex crispus
Origin	Europe
Part used	Root
Dose	1 teaspoon per cup, taken once daily at night

BULK LAXATIVES

Psyllium seed

Latin name	Plantago psyllium
Origin	Europe
Part used	Seed
Dose	1 teaspoon in 1/2 cup cold water once daily at night
Constituents	Mucilage, oil, sterols, bitter iridoids
Primary action	Bulk laxative
Secondary action	Nutritive
How it works	Psyllium mucilage swells up in the water and provides a soft, non-soluble fibrous bulk in the bowel. This stimulates peristalsis and is demulcent to the bowel wall. The oil in psyllium is polyunsaturated and contributes

some nutritive value.The iridoids are mildly bitter, so they are gently tonic to digestion.

Linseed

Latin name	Linum usitatissimum
Origin	Worldwide
Part used	Seed
Dose	1 teaspoon in 1/2 cup cold water, once daily at night
Constituents	Oil, mucilage, protein, cyanogenic glycosides, pectin, phosphates
Primary action	Bulk laxative
Secondary actions	Nutritive Healing
How it works	Linseed mucilage swells in water and provides a soft fibrous bulk which stimulates peristalsis. This relieves distension and promotes regular evacuation. Linseed also contains a high percentage of mono unsaturated and polyunsaturated oils (including linoleic acid). These are nutritive and help to maintain a healthy blood fat profile and increase healing of mucosal wall by contributing to cell structures. The protein is also nutritive. Pectin helps to bind fats, so preventing absorption, softening bowel content and lowering cholesterol levels. In addition to all these interesting effects, linseed oil provides building blocks for hormones and its cyanogenic acids are

centrally antispasmodic (acting on the brain). This is probably a minor effect as the quantity of this constituent is quite small. There has been no research into this aspect of linseed.

Doctors and chemists often supply other types of bulk laxative, which are based on the cellulose portion of bean husks such as isphagula and gums such as sterculia (karaya gum). These provide highly absorbent, insoluble fibre and often cause wind and bloating. They have no nutrient value, although karaya is demulcent if taken with sufficient water. Commercial preparations of these bulk laxatives often contain other medicines.

IRON TONICS

Oats	Nettle	Parsley	Watercress

These are foods which are regularly taken in our daily diet and do not have a specific medicinal dose. More iron-rich foods will be mentioned in the chapter on nutrition.

The iron in plants is not as easily absorbed as that in animal flesh, but herbs such as parsley and watercress contain a lot of vitamin C, which increases absorption of iron if taken at the same time (by as much as 60%). Alcohol also increases iron absorption, so tincture of oats and nettle may be used for this purpose. These and other herbs may be taken with a vitamin C rich drink such as orange or lemon juice. The extra iron provided by these herbs can offset losses due to slow internal bleeding, chronic diarrhoea or menstrual losses.

ANTI-SPASMODICS

Catnip	Meadowsweet	Wild yam
Chamomile	Parsley	Yarrow
Lemon Balm	Peppermint	

Catnip

Latin name	Nepeta cataria
Origin	Europe
Part used	Leaf
Dose	1 teaspoon per cup Tincture 4ml, 1-3x daily
Constituents	Volatile oil, bitters, tannins
Primary actions	Febrifuge Relaxant
Secondary actions	Carminative Anti-spasmodic
How it works	The volatile reduces bacterial fermentation in the bowel, so relieves wind and bloating. It acts directly on smooth muscle as an anti-spasmodic and some of its components have a relaxing effect on the brain. Tannins are also antibacterial and reduce sensitivity of the bowel wall. Parts of the volatile oil support this action by a numbing effect. Catnip is mainly known as a cold and fever remedy,

	but is useful in spasmodic bowel disorders.
Growing guide	Propagate by layering (burying sections of rhizome). Prefers sun, needs protection from cats!

Chamomile

(See Anti-inflammatories)

Lemon Balm

Latin name	Melissa officinalis
Origin	Europe
Part used	Leaf
Dose	1 teaspoon per cup 1-3 cups per day Tincture 4ml, 1-3 times daily
Constituents	Volatile oil, flavonoids, phenols, triterpenes, tannins
Primary actions	Relaxant Digestive tonic
Secondary actions	Anti-viral Anti-thyroid
How it works	The volatile oil has a central relaxing effect (on the brain) as well as reducing thyroid hormone stimulation of other systems. It also inhibits the growth of viruses such as herpes by giving a sort of repellant protection to the tissues and possibly penetrating viral coating. The phenols add to this effect and help to dispel bacteria in the gut. Triterpenes are bitter, so stimulate digestive secretions. Tannins astringe the wall of the gut,

alleviating diarrhoea.

Growing guide You will rarely have to resort to seed, nearly everyone has some lemon balm to give away. It seeds itself like mad, tolerates any soil and will grow in pots.

Peppermint

Latin name Mentha piperata

Origin Europe/world

Part used Leaf

Dose 1 teaspoon per cup
Tincture 4ml, 1-3 times daily

Constituents Volatile oil, bitters, tannins, flavonoids, azulene, phenols, isovalerates, methyl acetate

Primary actions Carminative

Secondary actions Digestive stimulant

How it works Methyl acetate in the volatile oil numbs GIT linings, relieving pain and allowing calmer movement. Tannins and phenols reduce bacterial ferment, relieving wind and bloating. Azulene is also noted for its antibacterial effect. Bitters stimulate digestive activity and isovalerate is mildly relaxant, acting on the brain. Flavonoids make blood vessels less fragile, so reduce inflammatory swelling. You can see from the complex chemistry of this plant that using the essential oil would not be as effective as using the whole plant or its equivalent.

Growing guide Easily grown from seed in a container. Keep

away from other varieties of mint as they cross-pollinate very easily which gives a weaker type of volatile oil.

Parsley

Latin name	Petroselinum crispum
Origin	Europe
Part used	Leaf
Dose	Mainly used as a food item, 10g fresh leaf could be taken on food as a regular part of weekly diet (on alternate days).
Constituents	Volatile oil, coumarins, flavonoids, minerals, vitamin C, A
Primary actions	Anti-spasmodic Diuretic
Secondary actions	Nutritive tonic
How it works	The volatile oil is antibacterial and anti-spasmodic, acting directly on the GIT muscles. Coumarins are also directly anti-spasmodic. The flavonoids are diuretic (increase elimination of water via kidneys). Parsley is rich in iron, vitamins A and C, calcium, phosphorus (which gives the bad smell when parsley rots) and other trace elements. It is best added fresh at the end of cooking.
Growing guide	Difficult to germinate, needs heat and well-drained soil. A cloche over seeds will usually do the trick.

Wild yam

(see Anti-inflammatories)

Yarrow

Latin name	Achillea millefolium
Origin	Europe
Part used	Leaf and flower
Dose	1 teaspoon per cup Tincture 4ml, 1-3 times daily
Constituents	Volatile oil, bitters, tannins, isovalerianic acid, salycic acid, sterols
Primary actions	Circulatory tonic Anti-spasmodic
Secondary actions	Digestive tonic
How it works	The volatile oil is anti-spasmodic, acting directly on GIT muscle and on the brain. Isovalerianic acid also has a relaxing effect on the brain. Yarrow is quite bitter, so stimulates digestion. Salycic acid is anti-inflammatory and pain-relieving by a central action. Tannins support this action by direct effect on the bowel wall and reduce bacterial levels. Yarrow's anti-spasmodic effect extends to blood vessel walls, so it helps to lower blood pressure. The sterols may be involved in relieving menstrual cramps.
Growing guide	The medicinal sort does not grow well in gardens as it likes to be surrounded by the complex biodiversity of meadow grassland.

RELAXANTS

Betony	Limeflowers	Vervein
Chamomile	Skullcap	Wild yam
Kava-kava	St John's wort	
Lemon balm	Valerian	

Betony

Latin name	Stachys betonica
Origin	Europe
Part used	Leaf
Dose	1 teaspoon per cup Tincture 4ml, 1-3 times daily
Constituents	Alkaloids, tannins, bitters
Primary actions	Nervine relaxant
Secondary actions	Digestive tonic Astringent
How it works	The alkaloids are relaxant by acting on the brain. Tannins are astringent throughout the GIT, reducing bacterial infection, pain and aiding healing. This herb used to be recommended as a cure for drunkenness, although there are no modern trials of this effect!
Growing guide	Prefers shady, damp soil.

Chamomile

(see Anti-inflammatories)

Kava-kava

Latin name	Piper methysticum
Origin	South Sea Islands
Part used	Root
Dose	1 teaspoon per cup, 1-2 cups per day Tincture 3ml, 1-2 times daily
Constituents	Pyrones, piperidine alkaloids, glycosides, mucilage
Primary actions	Relaxant Anti-depressant
Secondary actions	Anti-spasmodic Diuretic
How it works	Not much is known about the actions of kava-kava, though research is increasing as it becomes popular.The pyrones and piperidines act centrally (on the brain) to reduce sensitivity to pain. Applied topically it is rubefacient and numbing. It also has a reputation for relieving fatigue, so in some books it is referred to as a stimulant. It is best to view it like alcohol, relaxing and stimulating at the same time, with some effects of intoxication at high doses.
Growing guide	Not possible in the British Isles.

Lemon Balm

(see Anti-spasmodics)

Limeflowers

Latin name	Tilia europaea
Origin	Europe
Part used	Leaf and flower
Dose	1 teaspoon per cup, 1-2 cups per day Tincture 4ml, 1-3 times daily
Constituents	Volatile oil, flavonoids, phenols, mucilage, tannins
Primary actions	Relaxant Lowers blood pressure
Secondary actions	Increases sweating Anti-spasmodic
How it works	The volatile oil reduces brain's sensitivity to pain messages. Mucilage soothes stomach and gut wall and flavonoids make blood vessels less fragile. Phenols are antiseptic and diaphoretic (increase sweating), which induces dilation of blood vessels. The overall effect is to calm and lower blood pressure. Limeflowers is a particularly nice tasting tea.
Growing guide	Too large for the average garden, a most magnificent specimen can be seen at Kew Gardens in London.

Skullcap

Latin name	Scutellaria laterifolia
Origin	American
Part used	Leaf
Dose	1 teaspoon per cup, 1-2 cups per day Tincture 3ml 1-3 times daily

Constituents	Flavonoids, glycosides, iridoids, volatile oil, tannin
Primary actions	Relaxant
Secondary actions	Anti-spasmodic Possibly anti-inflammatory
How it works	Little is known about the active constituents of American skullcap as most research is based on a Chinese variant. We rely on the tradition of use for our knowledge of its actions. The anti-inflammatory effect is present in the Chinese variety and it is very likely that both varieties have the same constituents. American Skullcap is noted for its central (brain) calming effect, flavonoids stabilise blood vessel walls and contribute to its mooted anti-inflammatory effect, as well as mildly increasing the elimination of water via the kidneys. It has a long traditional use for neurological diseases such as epilepsy and motor neurone diseases.
Growing guide	Prefers damp soil, sow under glass and plant out in early summer in a warm, damp spot (pond-side, bog-garden).

St John's Wort

Latin name	Hypericum perforatum
Origin	Europe
Part used	Leaf and flower
Dose	1 teaspoon per cup, 1-2 cups per day Tincturn 5ml per day

Constituents	Essential oil, hypericin, hyperforin, flavonoids, tannins
Primary actions	Anti-depressant Relieves anxiety
Secondary actions	Relaxant Topical pain relief
How it works	The whole herb produces a calming and uplifting effect which reduces the perception of pain as well as inhibiting painful processes such as spasm and inflammation. None of the individual constituents have proved to be effective on their own. The oil applied topically is anti-inflammatory and pain-relieving. Useful for neuralgia, shingles and earache.
Caution	A recent research trial suggests that St John's Wort may make the liver destroy some drugs. This could be important for medicines whose dose has to be very precise, such as anti-epileptics, immune suppressants, heart regulators and HIV treatment. This research was based on a standardised type of St John's Wort where extra hypericin had been added. No trials using non-modified St John's wort have shown such results, but we now advise patients taking any of the medicines above to avoid this herb. It is perfectly safe to use externally with any medication except drugs designed to make your skin more sensitive to sun (some psoriasis sufferers take these).

Growing guide	Easy to sow direct in spring. Will tolerate most soil.

Valerian

Latin name	Valeriana officinalis
Origin	Europe and Asia
Part used	Root
Dose	1 teaspoon per cup, one cup per night Tincture 2-5ml nightly
Constituents	Valerianic acid, alkaloids, glycosides, tannins, choline, flavonoids, valepotriates, iridoids
Primary actions	Relaxant/sedative
Secondary actions	Anti-spasmodic
How it works	Valerianic acid and valepotriates reduce exciteability of brain and feelings of anxiety. Best used at night as it is on the borderline between relaxants and sedatives. Flavonoids are mildly diuretic (increase water elimination).
Growing guide	Sow directly in a sunny spot with damp soil in early spring.

Vervein

Latin name	Verbena officinalis
Origin	European
Part used	Leaf, flower
Dose	1 teaspoon per cup, 1-3 cups per day Tincture 3ml, 1-3 times daily
Constituents	Glycosides, iridoids, bitters, volatile oil, alkaloids, mucilage

Primary actions	Relaxant Bitter digestive tonic
Secondary actions	Anti-depressant Anti-viral Febrifuge
How it works	Not all actions are clearly understood. Bitters stimulate liver and digestive secretions, unknown constituents act on the brain to reduce sensitivity to pain and increase feelings of well-being. These are probably found in the volatile oil, which is responsible for the anti-viral effect, acting as a repellant in the tissues of the body. This is known as the 'constitutional effect' which French aromatherapists call the 'terrain theory'.

Wild yam

(see Anti-inflammatories)

Note

There are several relaxants and anti-spasmodics which are not available over the counter, but can be obtained by consultation with a qualified medical herbalist. These include lobelia (for bronchial spasm and muscle cramps), belladonna, and henbane (used mainly for kidney colic). See page 140 for medical herbalists.

CARMINATIVES

Angelica	Coriander	Juniper
Aniseed	Cumin	Lovage
Caraway	Dill	
Cardamon	Fennel	

The most well-known carminatives can be studied together as a group, as they are so similar in constituents and actions. They reduce bacterial fermentation in the GIT, and relieve muscle spasm and wind.

Aniseed, caraway, cumin, dill, fennel

Dose	1 teaspoon per cup Tincture 4m, 1-3 times daily
Constituents	Volatile oil, coumarins, phenols, flavonoids
Primary actions	Carminative
Secondary actions	Antibacterial Astringent
How they work	The volatile oil acts directly on bowel muscle to relax it and reduces sensitivity, giving some pain relief. Coumarins contribute to the anti-spasmodic action. Phenols and parts of the volatile oil reduce bacterial ferment which relieves wind and bloating. Flavonoids are diuretic, which is a helpful side-effect of these seeds.

Other common carminatives

The following are widely used in cooking and teas in the same dose as the carminative seeds above:
Angelica
Cardamon
Coriander
Juniper
Lovage.

ANTI-INFECTIVES

Pungent	Aromatic	Mixed effects
Cinnamon	Rosemary	Garlic
Clove	Sage	Myrrh
Galangal	Savory	Wormwood
Ginger	Thyme	
Horseradish		
Mustard		

Pungent anti-infectives

These pungent spices contain strong antibacterial elements in their volatile oils which relieve infection, wind and distension. They stimulate surfaces with which they come in contact and so increase peristalsis and digestive secretions. This also causes dilation of small blood vessels, which enables greater delivery of blood and transport of nutrients from the intestines. They are generally taken as food and may be used freely in cookery.

Aromatic anti-infectives

These aromatic herbs contain volatile oils which are mildly irritant to the surfaces they contact (less so than the pungent spices) so are safe to use with delicate digestive systems. They improve circulation by the same effect and increase peristalsis. Some components of their oils relax GIT muscle directly. Their bitters stimulate digestion and phenols are anti-bacterial, helping to relieve fermentation and wind.

Mixed effects

These are anti-infective herbs whose use goes back to antiquity. They display mixed effects.

Garlic

Latin name	Allium sativum
Origin	Europe/world
Part used	Bulb
Dose	1-3 cloves daily
Constituents	Volatile oil, pungent sulphur compounds
Primary actions	Anti-infective
Secondary actions	Anti-thrombotic
How it works	One of the sulphur compounds, alliin, has a range of of antibiotic activity comparable to broad spectrum antibiotics prescribed by doctors today. Garlic's volatile oil is a complex mix of pungent and aromatic constituents. It stimulates the linings of the GIT to increase peristalsis, but it is surprisingly well tolerated by individuals with sensitive digestion.

Growing guide	Plant out in autumn to produce bulbs the following summer.

Myrrh

Latin name	Commiphora molmol
Origin	Africa
Part used	Resin
Dose	2g resin piece to suck, or Tincture 2 -4ml, 1-3 times daily
Constituents	Resin, volatile oil, bitters,
Primary actions	Anti-infective Healing
Secondary actions	Astringent Carminative
How it works	The volatile oil is antiseptic and carminative. The resin 'smothers' bacteria by direct contact and soothes the surface it is applied to. Bitters stimulate better digestion via the liver and secretory linings of the gut.
Growing guide	Not suitable for cultivation in Britain.

Wormwood

Latin name	Artemisia absinthum
Origin	Europe
Part used	Leaf
Dose	1/2 teaspoon per cup Tincture 2ml, 1-3 times daily
Constituents	Volatile oil, bitters, flavonoids, phenols, tannins, coumarins
Primary actions	Bitter tonic

Anti-parasitic

Secondary actions Anti-infective

Carminative

How it works Wormwood's volatile oil is immensely complex, containing chemicals from many groups of plants such as Pine, Chamomile, Cedar, Mint and Rosemary. These are strongly anti-infective and act with other compounds specific to wormwood in removing intestinal worms safely and without griping. The same chemicals are anti-bacterial throughout the GIT, and the phenols and tannins contribute to this effect. Tannins also protect inflamed surfaces and coumarins ensure relaxation of the bowel muscle, acting directly on it. Wormwood is intensely bitter, so increases digestive secretions which improves breakdown and absorption of nutrients. Wormwood is an effective herb for bowel problems which appear to become chronic after an infection.

Growing guide Easy to grow but rather a weedy looking herb.

DEMULCENTS

Linseed	Psyllium seed	Slippery elm
Marshmallow root		

Linseed, Marshmallow root, Psyllium seed, Slippery elm

Dose 1 teaspoon to 1/2 cup water, 1-3 times daily

How they work These contain mucilage which is a kind of starch released by soaking in cold water. This provides a protective coating over the entire digestive system and contributes a mild bulk laxative effect.

DIGESTIVE TONICS

Boldo	Dandelion root	Lemon balm
Chamomile	Hops	Vervein

This group includes pungent spices and aromatic bitters mentioned in anti-infectives above, as well as relaxing bitters and bitter tonics.

Boldo

Latin name Peumus boldo

Origin S. America

Part used Leaf

Dose 1 teaspoon per cup
Tincture 4ml, 1-3 times daily

Constituents	Bitter alkaloids, volatile oil, flavonoids
Primary action	Bitter tonic
Secondary action	Diuretic
How it works	Boldo is a pleasant-tasting, aromatic tea. Mild bitters stimulate digestion and volatile oil is carminative. The flavonoids are diuretic and may account for its reputation as a slimming tea.

Chamomile

(see Relaxants)

Dandelion root

Latin name	Taraxacum officinalis radix
Origin	Europe
Part used	Root
Dose	1 teaspoon per cup Tincture 4ml, 1-3 times daily
Constituents	Bitters, phenols, inulin, vitamin A
Primary actions	Bitter tonic
Secondary actions	Diuretic Urinary antiseptic
How it works	Bitters stimulate digestion, phenols are antibacterial and inulin is a sweet-tasting diuretic. Dandelion has a pleasant bitter-sweet taste which makes it suitable as a caffeine-free coffee substitute. Its all round use has led to it becoming the emblem of the National Institute of Medical Herbalists, whose members keep the traditions of British herbal medicine alive.

Hops

Latin name	Humulus lupulus
Origin	Europe
Part used	Strobiles (flower-like growths)
Dose	1 teaspoon per cup, 1-2 cups per day Tincture 2ml, up to three times daily
Constituents	Volatiles oil, bitters, tannins, oestrogens, flavonoids
Primary actions	Sedative Bitter tonic
Secondary actions	Diuretic
How it works	The volatile oil reduces nervous activity in the brain and reduces muscle spasm in the GIT. The bitters promote effective digestion and the flavonoids are diuretic – they incrase the elimination of water. Tannins help to reduce inflammation of the gut wall.
Caution	Avoid in depressive illness.
Growing guide	A beautiful climbing perennial plant grown from root cutting or layering.

Lemon balm

(see Relaxants)

Vervein

(see Relaxants)

5

Growing and making your own herbal remedies

You can prepare herbs in a wide variety of ways to bring relief in IBS and colitis.

Types of herbal preparation

Oral remedies

Oral remedies are swallowed in measured doses. They include:

- teas
- tinctures
- syrups
- pills.

Topical remedies

Topical remedies are applied to the skin and include:

- creams
- oils
- baths
- plasters and poultices.

Oral remedies

Teas or tisanes

Teas, also called tisanes, can be made directly from dried herbs.

- Leaves and flowers require five minutes steeping in freshly boiled water. Always place a saucer or cover on the cup to keep in valuable aromatic ingredients. This is known as an **infusion**.
- Roots, barks, seeds and berries need boiling for five minutes in a covered pan. This is called a **decoction**.

The usual dose is one rounded teaspoon per cup (about 4g to 165ml). Regular use means one or two cups per day for several weeks. Infusions and decoctions can be drunk cold, and any flavouring can be added after steeping or boiling.

- To make an infusion steep cut leaf or flower for 5-10 minutes in boiling water.
- To make a decoction boil cut root or bark for 5-10 minutes on the stove.

Many people ask if the dosage of dried herbs should be different from fresh herbs. As the loss of chemicals in drying may balance the greater concentration due to loss of water, it is best to simply use the same amounts whether fresh or dry. Some herbs such as lemon balm, chamomile and basil, taste better when fresh and are slightly more effective, but most herbs keep their medicinal qualities very well if dried carefully. Roots and barks often improve their taste with drying as they lose their acrid components and become sweeter.

Measurements

1ml = 1g
1 teaspoon = 5ml
1cup = 165ml
Tinctures are usually 1:5, or one part herb to five parts alcoholic liquid.

Doses for adults

Adults will usually require one to three cups a day of herbal teas (whether infused or decocted), using one teaspoon of herb per cup.

Adult doses of tincture vary according to the herbs used in them. Usually half a teaspoon of single herb tinctures, three times daily, is required. With great care you can get 80 drops onto a 5ml teaspoon, so you can work out your dose that way too, and use the formula given above to calculate a child's dose. The amount of alcohol is negligible, but you can add the remedy to hot water and allow some of the alcohol to evaporate if you wish. Elderly people may require different doses, as body weight falls or if digestion isn't as good. One should start with a lower dose and work up if required.

Doses for children

Children require smaller doses. There are some formulae

which can be used, based on a child's age. For example, divide the child's age by twenty to give the proportion of an adult dose, i.e. 6 (years) divided by 20 = 3/10 adult dose. You also have to take into account the child's body weight, giving less if a child is underweight for his/her age.

Common doses for teas are; a tablespoon of tea to a child under 5, half a cup for a child from 5 to 10 years and a full cup from 11 years onwards. Beatrice Potter seems to agree, as Peter Rabbit was given a large spoonful of Chamomile tea after he had over–eaten in Mr McGregor's garden!

Making your own formula

You can combine herbs in tincture or tea form to obtain a mixture of effects which will suit your individual needs. Start by choosing the actions that you want – for example relaxant, pain relieving, hormonal, and look for herbs which provide them. It is best to include no more than three or four herbs in one mixture, and with careful selection you can choose herbs with more than one action to match your requirements.

If you are using dried or fresh herbs to make teas, you should choose herbs which require the same sort of preparation (remember that roots, barks and seeds need boiling, leaves and flowers need infusing). You will only need one teaspoon of your mix because herbs act synergistically as you have learnt already.

Tinctures

These have become very popular in Britain, both among herbalists and consumers. They are made by soaking herbal material, finely chopped, in an alcoholic liquid about 70% proof. This could be brandy or vodka. Generally, you use one part herb to five parts liquid, so 100g to 500ml. Chop the herbs as finely as possible and cover with the alcohol. Turn, shake or stir every day for ten days. This is to ensure that every particle of herb is in contact with alcohol, otherwise moulds may develop. After ten days strain and squeeze out the remaining 'marc' through a clean piece of material. Keep the tincture you have made in a dry bottle with a tight stopper.

This can be used in place of herbal tea. Each teaspoon of tincture generally gives the effect of a small cup of tea. Sometimes herbal constituents are extracted better by alcohol, so it is a useful way of preserving herbs. In the past wines and vinegars were used. Their trace is found in the nursery rhyme Jack and Jill where Old Dame Dob did mend Jack's nob with vinegar and brown paper.

It is obvious that these are much bigger doses than is often suggested on over-the-counter tincture bottles, where the manufacturer is more concerned with keeping the price and profit margin at an attractive level. Tinctures are more expensive than teas, and you should expect to pay between £3 and £5 for a week's supply.

Tincture of lemon balm
100g lemon balm
500ml vodka or brandy

Chop herbs finely, cover with alcohol, shake or stir daily for ten days, strain and bottle.

Herbal syrups

Herbs can be preserved in syrup but they are quite difficult to make as the proportion of sugar to herbal material is crucial. They frequently go mouldy, however carefully you measure. There are two methods, the first is the simplest but only keeps for a few days.

Syrup recipe 1
Place chopped herb and sugar in 1cm layers in a clean, dry jar, finishing with a sugar layer. Leave for one day. You will find a syrup has formed. You can shake the jar gently once a day until all the sugar has turned into syrup. This may take three days but you can use the product immediately.

Syrup recipe 2
Soak 4g of herb, finely chopped, in 56ml water for 12 hours. Strain and squeeze out the herbs. There should be about 45ml liquid. Add 90g sugar, stir over heat until dissolved, boil briefly, strain through a filter paper or cloth. You should have about 100ml syrup. This must be kept in a well stoppered bottle in a cool, dry, dark cupboard. The dose would usually be 1 teaspoon at a time

for children, and a dessertspoon from 11 years onwards.

Pills

These come in two main varieties: pills and capsules. In both cases, powdered herbs are used. Capsules are usually made of gelatine, although vegetarian ones can be obtained. Most are of a standard size, containing about 2g of herb. You can buy herbs ready powdered and fill your own capsules by hand. It's a very sneezy, time consuming business! Tablets are made by pressing powdered herbs into the required shape. You will need to add ingredients to make the dough stick together and the tablets hold their shape. Manufacturers usually use vegetable gums, but quite satisfactory tablets can be made at home using honey and arrowroot as binders. Pills can either be pinched off and rolled between the fingers or tablets cut by hand from dough rolled with a pin.

Buckwheat pills

2 tablespoons buckwheat flour
1 tablespoon arrowroot powder
4 teaspoons runny honey

Knead all ingredients together. Add more honey if required to achieve a malleable paste. Dust board with arrowroot, roll out, cut to shape, dry on paper overnight.

Topical remedies

There are several forms in which herbs can be applied to the outside of your body. This is known as topical application. You need to remember a little bit about skin to understand how herbs reach their target when used in this way.

The skin

Skin has several layers designed to keep water in (you suffer dehydration quickly if large areas of skin are broken) but allow moisture out when required to cool the body down by evaporation. It is covered with a cornified layer (dead cells) and wax. Blood vessels are very close to the surface, and they dilate when we are hot to allow heat out by convection. They also dilate when we are emotionally stressed, so we flush with anger, embarassment or affection. These blood vessels can constrict to conserve heat, and sometimes when we are very angry or upset we become paler than our usual colour.

Fat underneath the skin keeps heat in by insulation and protects some areas from pressure (famously the bum!). Muscle is found underneath linings below the fatty layer. If you want to reach muscles, your topical applications must somehow get through the wax, cornified layer, fat and muscle linings first. Oily preparations do penetrate through these layers to some extent.

One way of increasing penetration is to soak the skin in water for a while. This can be done in the bath, in a steam room, or on small areas with a poultice or plaster. Belladonna plasters for back pain could still be bought in the chemist's until a few years ago. Most people have heard of anti-smoking and hormone patches. These use the same principle. Back to Old Dame Dob and her vinegar on brown paper!

Four ways of increasing absorption through the skin:

- bath
- steam
- poultice
- plaster.

Creams

Creams are more complicated to make. It would be easier to choose a favourite bland cream over the counter and add aromatic oils or tinctures as you wish. If you want to try a cream, try the following recipe.

Rosemary cream

8 parts oil
1 part beeswax
a few drops essential oil

Gently heat oil and beeswax together in a bowl, set in a pan of water. When wax has melted, add essential oil and pour into pots immediately.

Greasy ointments like this are generally not considered to be good for skin conditions such as eczema, where they inhibit healing and trap heat, but they are suitable for applying as muscle and joint rubs. Their advantage over liquid preparations is that they don't drip on your carpet.

Massage oils

This option is useful if you want to use herbs from your garden. Simply pick a handful of fresh herbs, chop finely and cover loosely with any oil – almond, olive or even sunflower oil. Place the bowl of oil and herbs in a pan of water and put the lid on. Heat until simmering and leave on the lowest possible heat for 1-2 hours. A slow-pot can give ideal conditions for making infused oils as it maintains a constant, very low simmering temperature. Spices can also be used in infused oils.

There are many essential oils available now which save you the time involved in infusing plants in oil. The easiest way to apply these is in a carrier oil such as olive, almond or coconut. A few drops to a tablespoon will suffice. You can add a dash of chilli or ginger! Massaging increases blood flow to muscles and breaks down the tension in them. This can help to relieve painful stomach cramps, where the superficial muscles have also become involved.

Baths

Essential oils can be added to the bath. Use a teaspoon of unscented bubble bath or a tablespoon of milk to act as a dispersant. Relaxing bath salts are based on the same principle and available commercially, although they don't smell as nice as genuine essential oils. The relaxing effect is limited, but a helpful contribution, especially at night before bed, and there are no side-effects.

Plasters and poultices

These are used to apply steady heat or continued absorption of pain relieving or relaxing constituents to joints or muscles.

Plasters are made by melting one part of beeswax and two parts of vegetable oil, adding tincture or essential oil at the last minute. Soak a suitable sized cloth in the mix and spread out on a tray to cool and firm up. Apply to the body and cover in plastic or cling film (or paper!) and tie on with a bandage or some tight garment. The most common use is application to chest, back, abdomen and forehead. You could add a hot water bottle or hot towel wrap for extra comfort.

Poultices are similar to plasters, but consist of a 1cm thick layer of fresh or macerated herbs applied to the skin and covered with a piece of material. This was the earlier form of a plaster, but can still be immediate and effective.

Choosing herbs

Identifying herbs in the wild

It is important first of all to know that you have the right plant. Some botanical families include poisonous and edible plants which look very similar and can only be distinguished from each other by fine botanical detail, like hemlock and valerian which have subtle differences in stem and flower colouring. You could buy a field botany guide, as identification of plants is a great hobby, but it would be wiser not to select your remedies from the wild if you are a complete beginner.

Fortunately many of the most important medicinal herbs are garden favourites such as thyme, sage, rosemary, lemon balm and peppermint. Most people recognise them and they are pretty unmistakeable. Even where there are different varieties such as the thymes and mints, they have the same aroma and characteristics. It is better to choose the original sort for medicinal purposes rather than a variety because it may be a more reliable source of the chemicals that you need for your remedy.

Choosing herbs

There is a system of naming plants which gives each one two Latin names- the family name comes first and has a capital letter, the individual name comes second written in lower case. The meaning is reversed in Latin, for example *Thymus vulgaris* means common thyme. This is the one you would use for cough medicine. Other types, such as *Thymus aureus* (golden thyme) or *Thymus serpillus* (creeping thyme) will do no harm, but they don't have as much aroma – in fact they put most of their energy into looking pretty! The same can be said for the many lovely varieties of achillea – a cottage garden flower related to yarrow (*Achillea officinalis*) The word *officinalis* in a plant's name means it was known to be used medicinally in the seventeenth century or before. You will need to specify both names when you are buying seeds or plants from nurseries. Addresses of reliable firms are given on page 139.

Growing herbs

Many of the herbs mentioned in this book can be grown in British gardens, some can be grown in pots or on window ledges. Growing herbs is a very relaxing and rewarding hobby. Although most aromatic herbs originate in the warm Mediterranean countries, they will do fine in a sunny spot in any garden soil, even on London clay. They do prefer well drained (slightly dry) soil, so adding grit and compost will help them along.

If you are growing from seed you will need to start them off in pots first on a window ledge or in a greenhouse. To sow seeds really successfully, you should buy John Innes compost number 1. This contains lots of sand and fine grit, so that water runs through quickly and the seed doesn't sit in its own tiny puddle of water, which causes a fungal growth gardeners call damping off.

When you have a small stem with two leaves pull it up gently and plant in a pot with John Innes number 2 compost. This has more soil, so that fine roots can spread and take in water – it also contains a little more nutrient to feed the growing plant. When your plant is about 10 cm tall or has a few branches, it's time to plant it in a sunny spot or container, using John Innes number 3. John Innes is a type of compost, not a brand name, so you can ask for it at any garden nursery.

Planting out

Locate your herbs in the south west corner of your garden if possible. Herbs don't need feeding or watering once they have extended their roots into the garden soil (after about a week) but containers will need to be watered as they dry out continually. You can even grow herbs in hanging baskets. You can use multi-purpose compost, but you run a much greater risk of damping-off and losing seed before they even grow, which can mean a whole growing year lost. If your plants don't succeed in one spot in your garden, move them! Just dig up enough soil around the plant to ensure minimum root disturbance and put them in somewhere else. Experiment to see what works. There are plenty of herbs to choose from, so find one that suits your garden or space.

- choose a sunny spot
- add grit to improve drainage
- start tender plants under glass
- water pots and baskets daily
- move plants if they aren't happy.

Choosing the right part of the plant

It is important to know which part of the plant you need if you are going to make your own herbal remedies. Flowers, leaves, roots, bark and berries are commonly used but sometimes one part of a plant is edible whereas another part is poisonous. We eat the tuberous root of the potato but avoid the berries and we eat rhubarb stems but not the leaves. Comfrey root stores too many alkaloids which can damage the liver, whereas they are barely present in the leaf. It is common to find stems in with leaves in herbs sold over the counter, as it is difficult to separate them when preparing herbs on a large scale. If you are preparing your own you should take the trouble to rub the leaves off the stems as your remedy will be stronger without this inert woody matter.

Harvesting herbs

Choosing the right time to harvest is also important. It helps you to get the best quality of herbs in terms of the chemical constituents.

- Leaves are picked just before flowers develop.

- Flowers are picked as they come out.
- Berries as they become fully ripe, while they are still smooth and shiny.
- Bark and stem is stripped in the late spring from new branches.
- Roots are dug up in early autumn before the first frosts.

Pick on a dry day, and scrub roots immediately after digging.

Storing herbs

Most plants can be used fresh, but it is more convenient to dry them for use all the year round. The rules for drying herbs are:

- as cool, fast, dark and dry as possible, with as much air circulating around the individual herbs as can be allowed.

The best way for home preservation is to hang up small bunches of herbs, loosely tied, in a dark room or shed. A washing-line strung across the attic is ideal. Hanging up in the kitchen will cause most of the colour and aroma to be lost before they dry.

Large roots should be chopped before drying, as they will prove too tough for the knife otherwise. They can be spread out in a single layer on newspapers. The newspapers should be changed when they feel very damp.

Herbal material is ready to store when it is cracking dry. This is a matter of experience. Usually leaves will simply not leave their stems until they are thoroughly dry. Roots should snap briskly or fail to bend under pressure. Berries usually give a little under thumb pressure. They are slow to dry – moulds develop if there is too much moisture so gentle heat (airing cupboard level) is helpful.

When thoroughly dry herbs should be stored in cool, dark, dry, airless conditions because sunlight destroys colour, air removes flavour and water causes moulds. Tin boxes are ideal, however plastic tubs and glass jars are OK provided they are kept in a cupboard.

- Hang leaves on branches upside down.
- Spread roots out in a single layer.
- Dry as fast as possible in cool, dark, airy place.
- Ready when cracking dry.
- Keep in cool, dark, dry, airless conditions.

6

Using nutrition for a healthy digestion

Achieving a balanced diet

Nearly everyone agrees that what we eat affects our health. Most complementary health practitioners believe that our diet affects the way we experience diseases as well. In Britain research into food was started during World War II and was continued by the Ministry of Agriculture and Fisheries with help from the Medical Research Council. They produced guidelines on what people need to eat to make them healthy. These are called the **minimum daily requirements** and they cover the main nutrients needed by the human body. In America USDA (the United States Department of Agriculture) funds a similar programme and their books are widely used in Britain.

It is a mistake to look at single nutrients as being a cure for specific conditions, as almost all body processes require a broad range of nutrients to keep them running smoothly. Several vitamins are required to enable absorption and use of minerals such as calcium, zinc and iron, so taking single nutrient supplements is often a waste of time and may in fact upset the balance of some minerals, which may displace others or hasten their elimination from the body.

All human cells need sugar as a fuel to perform their vital functions. Muscle uses sugar for fuel as well as calcium and potassium to contract and relax. Salt (sodium) plays an essential role in getting calcium into muscle fibre cells and potassium is vital to maintain the correct amount of salt in the body. All these processes are dependent on each other and on a balanced state of nutrients in the body. This is the state of health which the herbalist tries to restore with herbal medicines and wholistic dietary advice. It is usual to divide food up into seven different categories and we should aim to eat something in each category every day.

You could use these categories to design a food diary or plan your eating for a week.

- **Protein** – cheese, meat, beans, nuts, fish
- **Starch** – bread, potatoes, pasta, roots, rice, grains
- **Vitamin A** – green, orange and yellow vegetables
- **Vitamin B** – meat, wholegrains
- **Vitamin C** – fresh fruit and green vegetables
- **Vitamin D** – fish oil and sunlight
- **Vitamin E** – wholegrains and seeds
- **Vitamin P** – also known as bioflavonoids – fresh fruit and vegetables
- **Minerals** – calcium, potassium, sodium, magnesium, zinc, phosphorus, found in vegetable and animal foods
- **Trace elements** – cobalt, copper etc , found in

vegetable and animal foods
- **Fibre** – indigestible parts of vegetables and grains
- **Fat** – butter, vegetable and nut oils, margarine.

Daily requirements for nutrients

These vary according to age and occupation (whether you have an active or sedentary job). Here we have taken the figures for sedentary workers. You can use these tables to understand information given on labelling of supplements.

- 1mg = one thousandth of 1g , 1µg = 1 millionth of 1g

	Men 35-64	Women 18-54
kcals	2,400	2,150
protein	60g	54g
calcium	500mg	500mg
iron	10mg	12mg
vit A	750µg	750µg
thiamin (vitamin B_1)	1mg	.8mg
riboflavin (vitamin B_2)	1.6mg	1.3mg
niacin (vitamin B)	18mg	15mg
vitamin C	30mg	30mg
vitamin D	10µg if no sunlight available	10µg if no sunlight available

Women's needs vary to a greater extent than men's because of changes taking place during pregnancy, breastfeeding, the monthly menstrual cycle and menopause. British guidelines suggest that women over

55 take fewer calories (1,900kcals) and less iron (10mg) daily. The lower iron intake is suggested because there will be no monthly losses due to menstruation and the smaller calorie intake reflects metabolic changes after the menopause.

American researchers give us figures for some of the other vital nutrients which apply to both men and women.

vitamin k	70-140µg
biotin (vitamin B)	100-200µg
pantothenin (vitamin B)	4-7mg
potassium	1,875-562 mg
phosphorus	700-800mg
sodium	1,100-3,300
chloride	1,700-5,100

Canadian guidelines complete the picture, with daily requirements for men and women between 25 and 49 and recommendations for the over 50s (blank means no change).

	Men	(over 50)	women	(over 50)
vitamin E	9mg	7mg	6mg	
folacin (vitamin B)	220µg		175µg	190µg
pyridoxine (vitamin B_{12})	2µg		2µg	
magnesium	250mg		200mg	210mg
calcium	800mg		700mg	800mg
iodine	160µg		160µg	
zinc	9mg		8mg	

It is interesting to note that Canadian researchers think we need a lot more daily calcium than do their British counterparts. This is because they recommend a much higher protein intake which causes greater loss of calcium from the body.You may need to take this into account when you are looking at labels on vitamin and mineral supplements.

Other minerals considered essential for daily nutrition are chromium, selenium, molybdenum, copper, manganese and fluoride. The intakes for these are generally very small figures – from .2 to .5µg. These are called trace elements.

The guidelines presented above are based on the amounts needed to stop you developing a deficiency condition, such as scurvy which develops when you don't get enough vitamin C. Some nutritionists think you need more than these if you have certain diseases, but this is a very undefined area, with lots of claims motivated by the desire to sell products. Although, as stated before, general health is achieved by eating a balance of all necessary nutrients, some are more clearly associated with digestive health than others. We will explore the role of these nutrients in maintaining healthy digestive organs in this chapter. In addition to creating a healthy balance in our diet we will focus on one or two groups of foods which are of special benefit to the digestive system and require some explanation. We will also look at the role of special diets for IBS and colitis including elimination diets.

Fibre

Fibre is a type of starch derived from plants which isn't absorbed into the bloodstream from the intestine. It is the basis of all bulk laxatives. It has two forms – **soluble**, such as pectin and gum, and **insoluble**, such as cellulose and lignin. Pectin is found in fruits such as apples, pears and plums, and in the peel of citrus fruits. Gums, such as guar and xanthan, are found in beans and are commonly used as an additive to ice-cream and yoghurts. Cellulose and lignin is found in vegetables and grains (wheatbran is of this type).

Soluble fibre

Soluble fibre lowers blood cholesterol levels by binding to bile acids, which are made from fats, helping their safe removal from the body. They may swell up in water and slow the movement of food through the intestine, so they can help the irritated bowel move at a normal pace and still aid evacuation. This is what herbalists call a balancing action.

Insoluble fibre

Insoluble fibre increases the movement of the bowels and prevents excessive muscular constriction of the empty bowel. This action protects against the formation of diverticulae (pouches in the gut wall). It is the most effective measure against this condition. Lack of fibre is the greatest cause of divertivculosis (formation of pouches). Insoluble fibre absorbs water and creates a bulky feeling in the intestine. This type of starch is non-calorific. So can help to reduce weight as part of a calorie-controlled diet. Foods containing insoluble fibre provide less sugar and demand less insulin, so help to moderate the high blood sugar levels which diabetics suffer. Some types of bran, such as that in oats, actually bind to cholesterol like gums. Wheatbran on the other hand, binds to vitamins and minerals and prevents their absorption. This effect is eliminated by the process of leavening bread with yeast.

The filling effect of fibre is useful for adults who need to lose weight, but it is not desirable in small children who have a small GIT and need more concentrated nutrition, although adequate fibre is essential to maintain normal bowel movement. Fruit is particularly useful here as it may help to reduce the craving for sweet snacks and is not drying in the bowel like bran. It provides essential vitamins and minerals and a gentle bulk laxative action with both pectin and insoluble fibre.

Daily fibre requirement

An adequate fibre intake for adults is considered to be 20-30g daily.

2g of fibre is found in:

- 1 piece of fruit (apple, pear, peach, banana)

- 1 slice wholemeal bread
- 3 tablespoons of oatmeal
- 1/2 cup of barley
- 1 teaspoon of wheatbran
- 1/2 stalk of broccoli
- 4 brussel sprouts
- 1 dessertspoon of beans (kidney, haricot)
- 2 tablespoons of peanuts
- 1 medium potato
- 2 cups of lettuce

You need to take in a number of these items to fulfil your fibre requirements. British government advertising slogans advise five a day. Beans are a very rich source of fibre and protein and should be eaten regularly.

Essential fatty acids (EFA's)

There are two essential fatty acids, linolenic and linoleic.These are components of fats which are mainly found in plants but also in very small quantities in meat. Wild meat, also known as game, contains far more EFAs than domestic animal meat. They are needed to make cell membranes, especially in surfaces which are constantly being worn away and replaced, such as GIT linings. The human body cannot make these fatty acids and cell membranes cannot be made from any other type of fats. They are part of the group known as polyunsaturated fats, which includes arachidonic acid (made in the body from linoleic acid) and eicosapentoic acid (from fish) This fish oil has beneficial effects on blood circulation but is not used to make cell membranes. It is possible that a deficiency in these essential fatty acids (also known as omega 3 and omega 6 acids) may contribute to inflammation of the GIT linings, as they might be unable to secrete protective mucus efficiently.

There are few established recommendations for EFA's. American dietary researchers recommend 6g of EFAs daily, from mixed sources.British authorities suggest between 2-10g daily.

EFA content of foods, g per 100g

	Linoleic	Linolenic
safflower oil	75g	.5g
wholemeal flour	59.4g	4.1g
barley	57.4g	6.1g
potatoes	56.5g	17.2g
green peppers	56.3g	12g
corn oil	50g	1.6g
soya beans	52g	7.4g
sunflower oil	52g	.3g
grouse	31.9g	30.3g
rabbit	20.9g	9.9g
chicken	13.5g	.7g
rapeseed oil	15.5g	10.5g

There are no figures available for hemp, evening primrose and borage oils which are reported to have higher linolenic acid levels than other oils, and are much vaunted as dietary supplements for all types of diseases. Rapeseed oil is also known as vegetable oil, it appears low in the list for linoleic acid but has the highest content of linolenic acid of all the common cooking oils. Linolenic acid is also present in useful quantities in green leaves and beans. It appears from this table that eating a mixed diet with plenty of vegetables, especially beans and greens, will supply an adequate amount of both essential fatty acids without needing supplementation.

To maintain a healthy digestive system it may suffice to add 5-10ml of vegetable oils as a salad dressing to a green salad and reduce your animal fat consumption by taking low fat milk, game or white meat (or no meat), reducing cheese consumption and choosing 'white' cheeses such as Wensleydale, Caerphilly, Stilton, Lancashire, Cheshire and goat's cheeses as these contain a lot less fat than other varieties.

How to increase EFAs in your diet without increasing calories

- eat salad every day with dressing (lemon and oil)
- eat potatoes and roots instead of pasta
- cook with vegetable oils, use gentle heat for frying
- use soft vegetable margarine instead of butter
- make cakes with vegetable oils instead of hard margarine
- eat beans in salads, soups and with meals
- eat five portions of vegetables and fruit daily.

In addition, dieticians from the American Heart Association recommend that fat should only represent 30% of your calorie intake. Several books show elaborate schemes of 'calorie exchange' which are quite difficult to follow. By weight fat gives far more calories than starch, so a simpler approach might be to think in terms of a tablespoon (15ml) of fat a day from all sources. This would mean thinking carefully about cakes and pastries, which contain 'hidden fat'. The average pasty contains 50g of fat in the pastry alone! Baking fat is hydrogenated, which converts polyunsaturated fats into saturated fats. These cannot be used for cell membrane building, and leave you no room for further fat intake from healthier sources.

Special diets for IBS and colitis

The herbal approach is to relieve symptoms in the GIT and restore the bowel to a condition in which all foods can be taken without problems. However, many patients in the herbalist's clinic present an acute phase of colitis, where diarrhoea and weight loss predominate. For these cases herbalists generally recommend a bland diet.

Bland diet

This includes eggs, fish, chicken, potatoes, cooked root vegetables and finely ground cereals and starches such as cornflour, arrowroot, rice. The foods to avoid in acute phases are crisp-fried, salty foods including cheese, alcohol, coffee and strong tea, nuts, pickles, raw fruit and vegetables, pulses. The last three cause distension due to lack of efficient digestive enzymes in this phase.

In chronic severe IBS this diet is maintained for longer, with the addition of gentle bulk laxatives such as psyllium seed, linseed (well soaked) and pectin. The following items are added to the bland diet: raw leaf vegetables, cooked pulses, raw fruits, coffee with meals. This is followed for several months along with herbal medicine, until all symptoms have disappeared. Preferred foods may then be reintroduced to the base of a healthy diet as outlined above.

Elimination diets

If you wish to discover if any particular food causes problems, you will need to eliminate it entirely from your diet for two months. In the case of milk and wheat you will need to plan carefully to maintain adequate calcium and energy. Taking a supplement may be appropriate here, as it may be a temporary measure. You must reintroduce eliminated foods after two months to see if they cause any reaction – this is known as a challenge.

Eliminating wheat requires careful attention to labels if you use any packaged foods. You may find that you lose weight, as most cakes and breads are made with wheat. You should be careful not to turn to sugary snacks when energy is running low, as these are highly calorific and generally empty of other nutrients.

The 'anti-candida diet'

This is a diet which requires complete elimination of all sugar and fermented products, including alcohol and yeast. However, it is often recommended for symptoms of distension and wind. It is unlikely that drastic elimination of sugar and yeast products from the diet will alter gut flora substantially. This is because all carbohydrates are reduced to simple sugars by the time they reach the gut and, as we have mentioned before, most 'supermarket' breads aren't made with yeast, which is a desirable food item because of its useful effect on phytic acid. There is no direct evidence that consuming yeast favours fungal invasion of the GIT, and few confirmed cases of intestinal candidal overgrowth, except in those who regularly take antibiotics. Very few of those who suspect candidiasis have had endoscopic investigation of the GIT to confirm it.

It is more likely that turning from white flour and sugar to complex carbohydrate (such as wholegrains, fruit and vegetables) would have a beneficial effect on gut flora, because of the improved peristalsis and better supply of vitamins which aid absorption of nutrients. A thorough case history most often reveals more complex origins of IBS and colitis, involving the emotions, diet, lifestyle, infections and other conditions. This is the type of multifactorial complaint for which herbal medicine is favourable.

7

Case histories

The remedies outlined in each case study consist of herbal tinctures given in equal parts unless indicated. Patients would take 1 teaspoon, three times daily, usually before meals.

Case 1 Wind, distension and thyroid problems

Mrs R was a 60 year old retired office worker who had recently had an operation to reduce an over-active thyroid gland. For a year before her operation she had suffered frequent loose bowel motions with gurgling sounds in her intestines, which had been first diagnosed as IBS then as the result of a thyroid imbalance.

About one week after her operation severe constipation set in, with distension, wind, nausea and belching. She could only pass one stool a week, even with strong laxatives, and she had noticed that they were an unusual light colour, almost white. She was in considerable discomfort, her abdomen was swollen and the area over her gallbladder was tender to touch. We considered the possibility of gallstones, hepatitis and under-active thyroid.

Mrs R agreed to contact her GP to arrange a further test

to check her thyroid function and a scan of her gallbladder. The immediate herbal priority was to relieve constipation and give 'antibiotic' cover for a possible infective cause. Mrs R took a spoonful of lemon juice (for vitamin C) and three cloves of garlic a day for three days. Her remedy contained herbs to relieve liver congestion, relax mental tension and gut muscle.

The remedy

- Holy thistle – liver regenerative, bitter tonic.
- Valerian – central relaxant.
- Lemon balm – anti-spasmodic, bitter digestive tonic.

Mrs R also took 5-10ml cascara nightly as a stimulant laxative. This relieved the constipation, producing softer stools, but she still complained of a sense of incomplete evacuation. When her blood test results came back it was discovered that her thyroid was not functioning at all, and she began a course of thyroxine which resolved her constipation and all other problems within a month. Mrs R continued to take her herbal remedy until the thyroxine was achieving its full effect and the GIT was back to normal. This took two more months. We discussed the wisdom of not assuming all bowel problems were due to IBS!

Case 2 Bowel problems in old age

Miss J was a lively 80 year old retired bookkeeper who had suffered abdominal distension and flatulence since her teenage years. She felt nauseous and had no appetite. Her constipation had become worse over the last ten years, with one small bowel motion every three days, although she used strong stimulant laxatives every day.

She had troublesome, unco-operative, bullying neighbours which caused her emotional stress, and she had taken major tranquillisers for ten years, although had taken none in the past two years. She lived alone, as her household companion had died some years ago, and she slept very badly.

Gentle pressure on her abdomen revealed hard swelling throughout the right ascending bowel and transverse bowel. A recent barium meal scan had eliminated tumorous obstruction so we had to assume that extensive impacted faeces were the cause of the swelling. The likely cause was chronic use of stimulant laxatives which prevented the natural stimulation of peristalsis by bulk.

Miss J's priority was to relieve discomfort and wind, and achieve a more substantial, soft stool. She also requested some help with sleep. Her remedy was designed to relax bowel muscle and relieve emotional tension, to soften faeces and improve circulation to the bowel wall. We felt that strong laxatives might continue to be necessary due to the very long period of their use and the natural atrophy of the bowel muscles.

The remedy

- Butternut – laxative.
- Wild yam – muscle relaxant.
- Lemon balm – nervine relaxant and bitter tonic.
- Ginger – (10ml in total) circulatory stimulant.
- Hops – bitter, relaxing tonic.

Mrs R also took a mixture at night which consisted of:

- Cascara – stimulant laxative.
- Aniseed – carminative.
- Valerian – sedative nervine.

This resulted in a larger stool being passed after three days, with additional use of her usual Sennacots from the doctor. Miss J continued to take this medicine for several months. Although her bowel movements did not change dramatically, the swelling in her abdomen reduced considerably and she felt less discomfort. Her sleep certainly benefited from the night-time mix.

Case 3 IBS and tension headaches

Miss E was 24 years old and training to be a masseuse, whilst working part-time in the advertising department of a newspaper. She complained of alternating constipation and diarrhoea, which had started two years before and occurred in two to three day cycles. She had sharp pains above her umbilicus, with gurgling noises. Miss E also described frequent headaches and irregular, painful periods. Her diet consisted of yoghurt for breakfast, cheese and lettuce sandwich (white bread) for lunch and meat, rice or pasta for tea. This provided her with almost no fibre. Her doctor had diagnosed IBS and her case history confirmed this, diarrhoea being a sequel to the irritation caused by constipation.

Miss E's priority was to prevent the frequent, urgent toilet visits, which were interfering with her job and training. The herbal remedy was designed to relax visceral muscle, balance hormones, improve circulation and relieve emotional tension.

The remedy

- Chilli – (8ml in total) circulatory stimulant.
- Chamomile – nervine relaxant and anti-spasmodic.
- Barberry – bitter tonic.
- Mint – carminative, pain reliever.
- Passionflower – nervine relaxant.
- Yarrow – anti-spasmodic, menstrual regulator.

Miss E also took Avens and Marshmallow in a tea once daily, changed to brown bread, added oats to her morning yoghurt and an apple to her midday snack. The herbal treatment brought an improvement in two weeks. She reported no gurgling sounds and bowel movements every day, with no constipation at all. She said that she felt calmer but had still not experienced a menstrual period since her last visit. With bowel symptoms largely relieved, more attention could be given to hormonal balancing over the next few months, which resulted in more regular periods.

Case 4 IBS, arthritis and stomach ulcers

Mr C was a 56-year -old music teacher. He had been suffering from pains in all his joints, especially his knees, for some time. He was using aspirin regularly for the pain in his knees, which were hot and swollen. He had had an operation to remove his inflamed appendix nine years before, but the symptoms of flatulence, distension and pain continued, with increasing sensitivity to foods. Mr C had experienced internal bleeding and vomited blood, so he was obliged to cease taking aspirin and other non-specific anti-inflammatory drugs (NSAIDs). Steroids had not relieved the swelling in his knees. He was anxious to return to work, as more time off would affect his pension. Coffee gave him heartburn and pain in his stomach area, so he supposed that he must still be ulcerated.

Mr C was concerned to treat his arthritis and GIT problems together. His remedy was designed to heal ulcers, reduce joint pain and relieve flatulence.

The remedy

- Celery seed – anti-inflammatory, diuretic

- Aniseed – carminative.
- Hops – bitter relaxing tonic.
- Comfrey – healing astringent.
- Meadowsweet – anti-inflammatory, healer.

Mr C gained complete relief from his digestive problems and became more mobile, with a lot less joint pain, after three months.

Case 5 Diarrhoea, stress and anxiety

Mr B was a 30 year old housing association worker. He complained of stress, anxiety and depression, which he attributed to his job, in which he was confronted daily by angry tenants and would-be tenants. He felt particularly bad in the evening and didn't want to go to work next day. He was often nauseous, was losing weight and had no appetite. He suffered from frequent diarrhoea and felt he could never be far away from a toilet. His intestines gurgled loudly and frequently during the consultation. Mr B described himself as a worrier and said that he had never been a big eater as a youth. He had been prescribed valium by his doctor, which he took at night. This enabled him to sleep but it had not brought any change to his digestive disorder. He was mainly concerned about his lack of appetite and weight loss and confessed to fearing that he had a serious bowel condition such as cancer. Mr B was happy to try a combination of relaxing and healing herbs, with digestive tonic action. He understood that his case history didn't suggest any obstruction or progressive worsening of symptoms, although we couldn't rule out inflammation, so he decided to defer re-visiting his GP until he had tried the herbal remedy.

The remedy

- Skullcap – nervine relaxant.
- Vervein – bitter tonic, relaxing nervine.
- Gentian – bitter tonic, anti-infective.
- Fennel – carminative.
- Avens – astringent anti-inflammatory.

This worked extremely well. All Mr B's digestive symptoms had disappeared by the end of two months. He resolved to look for a new job and didn't return to his doctor for further tests. After four months on this herbal mixture he progressed to drinking lemon balm and avens tea, once daily, to maintain relaxation and anti-inflammatory healing effects.

Case 6 IBS, stress and asthma

Miss F, a 35-year-old cashier, first consulted a herbalist for insomnia with alternating constipation and diarrhoea. Her bowel symptoms were much worse when she was stressed and a recent separation had triggered feelings of anxiety and depression. She said that she was beginning to suffer panic attacks (shortness of breath and dizziness) in crowded streets. She was visiting a psychotherapist weekly, which she thought was helping her to manage her feelings without using tranquillisers or anti-depressants.

Miss B hadn't noticed any pattern in her irregular bowel movements, but found that symptoms such as wind and colic subsided towards the evening. She mentioned that she had suffered from asthma since she was 20 and used a Ventolin inhaler one to three times daily. Her diet was based on refined carbohydrates (white bread, pasta) and cheese. She agreed to include more fruit and protein in her diet and to take a medicine as well as a tea. This consisted of relaxants and anti-depressants as we felt that her bowel symptoms were directly related to her nervous tension, which created muscular spasm.

The remedy

- St John's Wort – anti-depressant, relaxant.
- Cramp bark – muscle relaxant.
- Lemon balm – nervine relaxant, bitter tonic.
- Vervein – relaxant, liver tonic.

This produced excellent results after two months, with an elimination of panic attacks and a more regular bowel movement. Miss B also found that she didn't need her inhaler quite as much, and we discussed further herbal treatment for her asthma when she felt her bowel condition was quite stable.

Sources and resources

Nutrition – further reading

MAFF Manual of Nutrition (HMSO). A brief guide to the contents of major foods and dietary guidelines with daily requirements. This book was used by every home economics student and teacher from the 1950s until the 1980s when cookery and nutrition became design and labelling!

Identifying herbs – further reading

The Concise British Flora Publisher, W. Keble-Martin (Ebury Press). The author was a vicar who spent all his spare time painting wild flowers. This is a remarkable book which captures the essence of each flower and plant. Better than photos for identifying difficult to recognise subjects. Not easy to use, as the plants are arranged in families, but worth persevering.

Exercise

The British Wheel of Yoga, 25 Jermyn St, Sleaford, Lincolnshire NG34 7RU Tel: (01529) 303233. The main association for yoga teachers and those interested in yoga. Hatha yoga is the type which has most general application – it is yoga for health. This is mainly what you will find being taught in evening classes and lunchtime sessions. It consists of a series of tone and stretch exercises which have been developed over thousands of years in India. Most teachers include some exercises from other strands of yoga as these are more directly designed to relax the mind and are associated with meditation. Some people with strong religious faiths are afraid that yoga involves taking up a mystic religion. This isn't true – the meditations are designed to make you aware of your mind and enable you to empty it. They can be performed by members of any religious group.

Seeds

King's Seeds, Monk's Farm, Coggeshall Road, Kelvedon, Essex CO5 9PG. Tel: (01376) 572456. Previously Suffolk herbs, this is the only company in Britain selling a wide variety of wild flower and herb seeds.

Samuel Dobie and Son, Long Rd, Paignton, Devon TQ4 7SX. Tel: (01803) 696444. Dobie's Seeds sell a wide range of flower and vegetable seeds, with a good selection of culinary herbs.

Seeing herbs

The Chelsea Physic Garden, Royal Hospital Walk, (entrance in Cheyne Walk), London. Tel: (0207) 352 5646. (Sloane Square tube). Probably the best collection in Britain, begun in the seventeenth century, brilliant teas and cakes, exquisite pleasure to walk round. Open Sundays from 2pm and some weekdays. Run by volunteers (who make the cakes!)

Buying dried herbs and preparations

Alban Mills Herbs, 38, Sandridge Rd, St Albans AL1 4AS. Tel: (01727) 858243. *www.lsgmills@care4free.net*
A very large range of medicinal and culinary herbs and spices, creams, oils, syrups, tablets, toiletries and essential oils. Small amounts no problem.

Gardening

The Henry Doubleday Research Association, Ryton Gardens, Ryton in Dunsmore, near Coventry. The Association has its own seed catalogue, run by Chase Organics, and a magazine for subscribers which gives advice on organic gardening and news of organic projects in Britain and abroad.

Gardener's Question Time, 2pm, Sunday Radio 4, repeated in the day-time during the week, has been offering gardening advice from a panel of experts to live audiences for generations. *Gardener's World*, 8.30 BBC2, still offers a designer-free zone of real gardening.

Consulting herbalists

The National Institute of Medical Herbalists (NIMH), 56 Longbrook St, Exeter, Devon EX46AH. Tel: (01392) 426022. *www.btinternet.com/~nimh/*. Established in 1864 to promote training and standards in herbal medicine. It is the oldest body of professional herbalists in the world. Members train for four years to a Bsc in Herbal Medicine, which involves herbal pharmacology, medical sciences and pharmacognosy (the science of recognising herbal compounds and materials).

Representatives of the NIMH sit on government committees and are involved in decisions on the safety of herbal medicines in Britain and Europe.

Counselling and talking therapies

Self-help books are abundant. You will need to read more than one to get an idea of the different sorts of talking therapies.

Patient support groups

These are extremely useful for sharing problems and solutions. Ask in your local library for the *Directory of Associations* which contains all national associations and is updated annually. The current secretarial address for the Coeliac Association is listed there.

List of herbs within their applications

Anti-infectives

Cinnamon
Clove
Galangal
Garlic
Ginger
Horseradish
Mustard
Myrrh
Rosemary
Sage
Savory
Thyme
Wormwood

Anti-inflammatories

Chamomile
Comfrey
Fennel
Liquorice
Marigold
Meadowsweet
Wild yam

Anti-spasmodics

Catnip
Chamomile
Lemon balm
Meadowsweet
Parsley
Peppermint
Wild yam
Yarrow

Astringents

Agrimony
Avens
Bayberry
Bistort
Cranesbill
Tormentil

Carminatives

Angelica
Aniseed
Caraway
Cardamon
Coriander
Cumin
Dill
Fennel
Juniper
Lovage

Demulcents

Linseed
Marshmallow root
Psyllium seed
Slippery elm

Digestive Tonics

Boldo
Chamomile
Dandelion root
Hops
Lemon balm
Vervein

Iron Tonics

Oats
Nettle
Parsley
Watercress

Laxatives

Alder
Buckthorn
Butternut
Cascara
Linseed
Psyllium seed
Rhubarb
Senna
Yellow dock

Relaxants

Betony
Chamomile
Kava-kava
Lemon balm
Limeflowers
Passionflower
Skullcap
St John's wort
Valerian
Vervein
Wild yam

General Index